Cold Winter Nights

Cold Winter Nights

Another Month in the ER

Dr. S

Writers Club Press
San Jose New York Lincoln Shanghai

Cold Winter Nights
Another Month in the ER

All Rights Reserved © 2001 by Dr. S

Writers Club Press
an imprint of iUniverse.com, Inc.

For information address:
iUniverse.com, Inc.
5220 S 16th, Ste. 200
Lincoln, NE 68512
www.iuniverse.com

See also:
www.dr-s-md.com

Or write to:
Dr. S
PO Box 81
Plattsmouth, NE 68048

ISBN: 0-595-18504-5

Printed in the United States of America

This book is dedicated to my family.

Contents

Acknowledgements

Continuing thanks to the many health care professionals, and all the others that have contributed to the unique experience that is my life.

Introduction

"Another sip at the fire hydrant..."

It occurred to me, while I was writing the precursor to this book, "Hot Summer Nights: a month in the ER," that a follow-on might be appropriate. The original book covered a cross section of patients as seen in the warm summer months. We really do see a completely different mix of patients and disease in the winter, when the temperatures are colder. Some of these differences are as one would expect: falls on the ice, respiratory illness, and the like. Some of the differences are unexpected, as you will see. My goal is to attempt to provide a balance in this book to round out the experience of emergency medicine.

As in my prior work, I am attempting to provide a realistic representation of the Emergency Department, absent popular media's drama and hype. I try to cover typical cases and case management, as well as some of the thought processes that take place during patient evaluation. I also reflect on many of the issues that an emergency physician faces while working in this environment.

Unlike on television, the majority of Emergency Department cases are things that would normally be treated in a doctor's office, be it summer or winter. Whatever the reason, good or bad, patients present to Emergency Rooms. Federal law requires that they are all seen, evaluated, and provided appropriate stabilizing treatment. This is all a part of federal governmental regulation known as EMTALA (the Emergency Medical Treatment and Active Labor Act).

Emergency Medicine can be best described as long hours of boredom and frustration punctuated by minutes of sheer panic. Popular media tends to compress all of the crazy moments into a single story or episode. In reality, they are randomly interspersed throughout any given day, week, or month.

As in my first book, I try to capture the essence of what I see in a month of shift work in a small city Emergency Department. I feel that this is a more accurate reflection of emergency medicine in general; the bulk of Emergency Room visits across the country occurs in this type of facility rather than at a large regional medical or trauma center. I have worked at each type of facility and have found that the patient cross sections are similar with an important difference. Regional facilities act as referral centers and get clusters of cases that cannot be handled in smaller facilities. This is usually due to the lack of some specific local resource, such as a neurosurgical consultant, or in-house cardiac catheterization capability. Regional centers also don't see very common medical issues strictly because they are addressed by referring hospitals. An example of this is appendicitis. It's a fairly common affliction, but rarely makes it to the regional hospital.

The small city Emergency Department sees it all. They are typically the only facility in the city, and they usually provide medical care for a broad expanse of the surrounding rural area as well. This "catchment area" is often two or more times the size of the city the hospital serves.

As I have already stated, my goal in this book is to introduce as much realism as I can to a snapshot of the practice of emergency medicine. This may offend some folks, but that is a risk of the writing business. Though I may make some derogatory comments and the like, it is not that I bear any ill will towards others; it is usually because of the frustration of the moment. Similarly, there is a segment of the medical community that has a vested interest in maintaining an altruistic and idealistic perception of medicine among the public. Once again, to them I apologize in advance, and suggest they find another book to read.

Emergency Medicine is about medical cases, and so most of this book addresses cases. The vast majority of these cases are really very generic, and I cover them in that manner. Any information that might even remotely betray confidentiality is omitted. The reality is that such information would not really be germane to this book anyway. I attempt to capture the cases, their flow through the Emergency Department, the thought that goes into investigating them, the medical issues involved, and the final disposition. You will find that I often expound on the frustrations we face. These are real issues common to most facilities, and can provide interesting insights into the Emergency Department and their patients.

At this point I would also like to comment on the team that actually proves emergency medical care. This truly is a team affair, consisting of nursing staff, and a range of other ancillary personnel. The emergency physician directs them all. By no means does this mean that the physician is the "most" important team member. The reality is that each member contributes to the overall effort. The final effect is similar to many professional team sports, like football or basketball. However, the stakes are much higher (and the pay is quit a bit lower).

I would also like to speak a bit about the general state of health care delivery in this country. The United States, without a doubt, has the most advanced medical care available on the face of the planet. However, the mechanisms by which that care is administered and funded is woefully flawed. Nowhere is this more apparent than from the front lines of the Emergency Department. There are a number of trends that I have observed that highlight some of the major problems. These are not new and unexpected, andt are frequently talked about in the media. It's brought home much more forcefully, though, when you see it playing out every day.

A prominent trend is the growing number of uninsured. From my personnel experience, this seems to have ballooned over the last several years. A majority of these folks seek care in the ER because local doctors have no obligation to see them if they have no ability to pay for the medical services they use. As a majority of these folks are unemployed or underemployed, they are usually without adequate means to accomplish this.

Another key problem is with the insured, both the privately insured, as well as those on Medicare and Medicaid. The insurance structure isolates patients from the true costs (and many of the implications) of medical care. In addition, it facilitates a sense of "entitlement" in the patients and their family. There is a growing feeling among these groups, that they should be able to get maximum medical care, regardless of cost or benefit. In the Emergency Room setting, this has led to a huge increase in patient visits both for reasons of convenience and with the purpose of an agenda. There are no disincentives to this behavior. The explosion of Urgent Care facilities only exacerbates this reliance on "fast food" medicine, and the expectation of "no-wait" care.

When I speak of patient agendas, it's that I've seen a growing trend of patients presenting to the Emergency Room with the expectation of a very specific outcome, regardless of whether it is appropriate or not. This runs the gambit of folks wanting antibiotics for their viral head colds, to the demand for a head scan for the bruised forehead sustained by a child while playing.

Another real issue in health care, especially in the ER setting, is the perceived litigation risk. In this environment, everything we do is done with the ongoing specter of lawsuits. Perhaps as much as 80–90% of all testing and diagnostics are strictly to minimize potential medicolegal risk. When multiplied by the thousands of other hospitals around the country, this has got to total billions of dollars.

Well, what's to be done about all of this? We've already seen that any sort of sweeping change is a political hot potato. With health care expenditures in this country approaching $2 trillion annually, you can imagine that there are a lot of vested financial interests that want to maintain the status quo. Maybe it's going to take some catastrophic failure of the system in order for credible change to occur. I don't know. You don't have to look very far ahead to see a crisis looming. Think of all the baby boomers out there that are approaching retirement. They are all going to want only the very best that medical science has to offer, regardless of expense.

Just some things to think about...

So without much further fanfare, my counterpoint to "Hot Summer Nights."

Shift 1

"Fruits and nuts..."

Sunday—18 Hours

Midnight

It's another cold and windy winter day. The slate is cleared by the prior shift, but the parking lot is full and that, of course, is a bad sign.

For those of you who have not read my previous book, it might be helpful for me to once again describe the department. We are a full service Emergency Department that sees roughly 14,000 patients a year. The city has a population of roughly 30,000, and we have a catchment area of perhaps three times that. In the department, we have two urgent care rooms, three general-purpose rooms, a two bay trauma room, an outpatient surgery room, and a cardiac room. If necessary, we can recruit two additional urgent care rooms, plus the entire outpatient area of roughly six bays. We mix and match the rooms to meet the demand. Well, on with it...

I start with a 10-year-old white male whose brought in by his dad with a twelve-hour history of nausea and vomiting. He's been having cramping prior each bout of the vomiting. "He just can't keep anything down." The father is worried about dehydration. The kid had a

1

24-hour stomach bug about a week ago, and this is very similar. His exam is completely normal. Lab is ordered, and a Phenergan supposi-tory (an anti-nausea medicine) is given. We'll see what the lab shows, but I'm sure it will be normal...

Meanwhile there's a 25-year-old white female with sinus pressure and sinus drainage for several days. Of course she smokes a pack or two a day, and is not interested in quitting. She just finished a course of Augmentin (a broad-spectrum antibiotic), but is no better. She com-plains that she has to sit up at night to sleep because the sinus drainage and cough are so bad. She seems unwilling to make the asso-ciation that her heavy smoking is most likely a major factor in her recurrent sinus and respiratory illnesses. She asks for codeine based cough medicine so she can sleep. I put her on Levaquin (another broad-spectrum antibiotic), because it's what she's expecting, and Flonase (a steroid) nasal spray. I give her the cough medicine she wants and send her on her way. She needs to stop smoking, but it's that age-old adage about leading a horse to water and the like. It falls on deaf ears.

This is another point where I need to digress for those who hadn't read my previous work, "Hot Summer Nights: A Month in the ER." Hospital politics come into play throughout patient care delivery. The directive from hospital administration is to maximize customer service and minimize complaints. Somehow over the last several years, medi-cine has changed to what I call "McMedicine." Hospital administra-tion pressures the Emergency Department to give the patients what they want in order to minimize complaints. Of course, they also want us to minimize expenses and maximize revenues. This has obvious potential for a range of Catch-22s. The goal then becomes one of giving patients what they want or expect, as long as it does not grossly violate standards of care or good conscious.

I see a 74-year-old white male who has a myelodysplastic syndrome (a malignancy of the bone marrow that afflicts mainly the elderly). He's pretty much end-stage, but has absolutely no insight into the severity of his disease. His bone marrow is completely failing, and he's needing blood and platelet transfusions every week or so in order to stay alive. He's here with a hot, swollen, painful joint since the morning. Folks like this are at risk for just about everything, and so we'll have to check it all. I order x-rays and a range of lab tests. The two things that come immediately to mind are gout and septic arthritis.

Gout is a defect in the metabolism of nucleic acids, the genetic material that exists within cells. This includes both dietary nucleic acids, and those associated with cell death and cell turnover in our bodies. It can lead to excessive concentrations of the metabolic waste product, uric acid, within the joints in the body. It can crystallize producing inflammation and pain in these areas. Folks with malignancies are especially prone to this problem because they often have a high turnover of cancer cells.

Septic arthritis is what occurs if bacteria gains access to a joint space. This also leads to inflammation, pus formation, and ultimate destruction of the joint, if not treated promptly. Folks with malignancies do not have an intact immune system, and are more susceptible to this type of infection risk.

Except for the red, hot, tender joint, this gentleman has no other exam findings. We check several laboratory tests and get a x-ray of the joint for good measure. In the meantime he gets some Toradol (an anti-inflammatory) and some Demerol (a narcotic) for his 10 of 10 pain.

Something that gets a lot of press these days is pain and pain management. The general consensus is that doctors aren't very good at managing it. What the common wisdom doesn't take into consideration (with respect to the Emergency Room) is that a lot of folks are less than forthright about their pain. Unfortunately there is no objective measure of pain. There isn't a test we can do to establish the exact amount of pain a person is experiencing. This means that our measures are very subjective. The most common measure of pain in adults is to ask the patient to rank the pain on a scale of 1 to 10, lowest to highest. Of course, drug seekers are savvy to how we assess pain, and they usually insist that they have a pain at or well above 10 (the upper limit of the scale). The bottom line is that if we managed pain in the ER the way some of the current guidelines recommend, we would be the junkies local candy store.

The squad's out.. Sounds like a drunken kid being brought in for evaluation...

And it's a 14-year-old white girl who's pissed at the world. She's been drinking with friends, and is picked up by the local police. She is brought in for evaluation prior to being released to her mother. Listening to the nurse report, it sounds like a pretty dysfunctional family, but what else is new in our society? She's pretty well out of it, so I need to establish that she's not received a toxic amount of alcohol (or anything else). It is possible to die if you get too much. It takes about seven times the legal limit, and this is usually fairly difficult for the novice to do. I order some general lab, including a blood alcohol, a urine drug screen, and a pregnancy test. These are pretty much the standard types of things we look at in similar circumstances.

Well I've got some down time while we wait for the lab and what not. I have quite a bit a dictation left over from yesterday, so I work at getting caught up.

Okay then, where are we? The 74-year-old with the hot joint probably has a septic joint. His cancer is in full swing, and he hasn't got much more than two neutrophils (bacteria fighting white cells) to rub together. Nothing else really fits. He has almost no platelets as well, so we can't put a needle into the joint (he wouldn't be able to stop bleeding) to try and get a culture of any fluid that might be there. I chat with his regular doctor. He'll admit him and treat him empirically for the types of organisms that could be involved.

Our 10-year-old has a viral stomach bug as I expected. The lab is all normal. The Phenergan suppository we gave him calmed his stomach nicely, and he's now able to keep fluids down. We'll just treat him symptomatically, and let him follow-up as necessary.

Our intoxicated 14-year-old is sitting at just about twice the legal limit. She'll be a few hours sobering up, but there's no immediate danger. Surprisingly, we find nothing else on board. Frequently with these kids we get a smorgasbord of methamphetamine, marijuana, and the like. She goes home with her mom to sleep it off.

Meanwhile, back to my dictation…

The slate is clear, and I hear my bed a calling…

2:00 AM

Zzzz…

Wow, a whole 20 minutes…then I'm back into the fray.

I see a 20-year-old white female who awakened 15 minutes ago with a "heavy head and dry throat." She feels she is "going to come down with something." This has prompted her to race immediately to the ER. Is this weird or what? It takes a huge dose of reassurance to convince her that she is going to be fine. I send her on her way.

2:30 AM

Zzzz…

Gee, 30 minutes this time…

Next is a 48-year-old white female who is convinced she's dying, or at least she's acting like she is. She's had a fever, sore throat, cough, and body aches for a day. She's in the examining room with covers pulled completely over her head. She's got a low-grade fever, but otherwise has a normal exam. We'll do a few hundred dollars of therapeutic tests, but if we find anything I'll be surprised. I guess influenza is a possibility given the time of year, though she tells me she's had her flu shot this season. We'll see…In my mind, I am tempted to categorize her in the fruit and nut category. It's turning into that kind of night.

Oh lovely, we've also got a 79-year-old white male with diffuse lower abdominal pain for thirty minutes. By the time he presents his symptoms have resolved. He's had these symptoms off and on for 3 or 4 months. He's completely symptom free now, but wants to have it evaluated. Of course, this is just what I want to be doing at 3 o'clock in the AM. I order a set of abdominal films. If anything, it sounds like some gas, irritable bowel, constipation, or the like.

And the answer is…Our dramatic 48-year-old female has a normal chest x-ray and lab. She may have a bit of bronchitis, but only if you use your imagination. She wants to be in the hospital, but I don't have a good justification. I tell her this, and she is NOT happy at all. She wants her regular doctor called, but he's not on call and can't be reached. Tough! It's likely viral, but I put her on some Levaquin (an antibiotic) for good measure, some Tessilon (a cough medicine), and a few Vicodin (pain medicine). She can use her own inhaler as she needs. If she gets worse she can come back, or follow-up with her regular doctor.

Our 79-year-old just has a lot of gas. I find out that he's been abusing laxatives in his quest for a daily bowel movement. It's likely that the laxatives, in addition to the Milk of Magnesia his wife is giving him, is the source of his cramping. We'll stop all that and put him on some Sorbitol alone (a dietetic sweetener that works well to produce bowel regularity without the long-term side effects of laxatives). This way he can titrate his bowel movements without the side effects of these other agents.

Next in the queue is a 21-year-old white female with a "migraine headache" for two hours. Surprisingly, she tells me that Toradol (an anti-inflammatory) works best for her. We are so used to people telling us that nothing but Demerol (a big gun narcotic) will work. Toradol? I can do it! She also asks why she can't get Toradol in pill form to use at home? I can't think of a reason, so I'll give her some of that too.

Folks with supposed "migraine headaches" are frequent visitors to Emergency Departments around the country. The biggest problem is that so many of them are prescription drug addicts, or have been using narcotics for their headaches for so long that they've traded their migraine headaches for narcotic withdrawal headaches. We really only see most folks with true migraine headaches once or twice ever. They are the ones that actually follow-up with their regular doctor, and have their headaches managed outside the confines of the Emergency Department.

One last jab from our 48-year-old with cough and congestion is so typical of many folks we see. She just doesn't feel she can work this weekend, and so she wants a work excuse. Sure, why not? I give her the get-out-of-jail card she's looking for. With many of our visitors this is the sole reason they come to our department. This is especially true in communities with manufacturing businesses that require a doctor's note to be excused from working.

I often joke that we should just leave work releases in the lobby. It would dramatically reduce the number of inappropriate ER visits.

Pretty pathetic "emergencies" we're having this morning. I've had about enough. The Zzzz monster is looking over my shoulder and so...

4:30 AM

Zzzz...

Well about an hour this time. This night really has a case of sleep interruptus.

We've got an 85-year-old white male who had fallen three days ago and has rib and back pain. He's been taking Daypro (an anti-inflammatory) since the fall, and now he can't pee. I doubt that the medicine is what's to blame. When I talk with him further, he's actually been having problems with this for years. We do a bladder scan (a special ultrasound to measure the amount of urine in the bladder), and he does have about a quart of urine sitting in there. Then he's off to Radiology for a peek at his back and ribs.

6:00 AM

We also have a 25-year-old white male with a 10-hour history of "migraine headache." He's got his usual headache, and it's not responding to his Tylenol with codeine. His regular doctor's office is going to be open in another couple of hours, but apparently he just can't wait another minute. I give him one of my usual concoctions: Nubain (a non-narcotic pain medicine), Phenergan (an anti-nausea medicine), and DHE 45 (a migraine abortant medicine). He's feeling better pretty quickly, and is ready to go.

We get a call from one of the local nursing homes. We're going to be getting a 95-year-old white female who took a tumble. It must be shift change at the nursing home. We invariably get a majority of these patients at shift change. There are a lot of different reasons for this, but none are very good.

Well our 85-year-old with the rib and back pain has decided he needs to stay in the hospital. His x-rays don't really show much of anything except for an 85-year-old skeleton. I have a urinary catheter placed, and send a sample of his urine off to the lab to make sure he doesn't have an infection. Then we're back to waiting mode for a while...

Our expected 95-year-old shows up by squad. She is demented to beat the band and complains of pain throughout her arms and legs. She is so confused and agitated that this becomes veterinary medicine. We just x-ray everything that seems to hurt. We're going to have her glowing in the dark. In someone this age with a ground level fall, she could break just about anything (or nothing at all).

Meanwhile we get another demented 94-year-old white female in by squad from a different nursing home. She had fallen this morning and is having severe left hip pain. She's unable to bear any weight. She's also off to Radiology.

It turns out that our 95-year-old did some severe damage. She's broken her hip and her shoulder! A call goes out to her doctor, and the orthopedic surgeon. She's admitted and up to the hospital floor in a jiffy.

And what do you know? Our 94-year-old lady makes for a duet of busted hips. She also gets admitted and is whisked up to the hospital floor.

We've got a 21-year-old white female with low abdominal pain for the last day. She had been seen elsewhere yesterday, and was felt to have pelvic inflammatory disease (an abdominal infection usually caused by the sexually transmitted disease, chlamydia). She was empirically treated with appropriate antibiotics (Rocephin and Doxycycline), and was also put on Percocet (a pretty big gun narcotic). Despite this, she continues to have unremitting pain. This suggests that she may not have the right diagnosis. She indicates that she's had ovarian cysts in the past. She also still has her appendix. Either one, ovarian cyst or appendicitis, is a possibility. We get her comfortable with some IV Demerol (a bigger gun narcotic), and send her off for a CT scan of her pelvis. Regardless of the findings we'll call her regular doctor. A repeat visit like this is likely to warrant admission for further evaluation.

Emergency medicine has a lot of unwritten laws that can keep you out of court. If the patient comes back, and you don't have reason to think they're just a drug seeker or the like, you always do more to evaluate them than the last time. If you're still not sure what's going on, and the list of possibilities could include something threatening, then get them admitted, and let someone else make the call. Similarly, if you've got a patient who is crashing fast, and you don't have a clue what's going on, then two rules apply: 1.) Spread the wealth. 2.) Spread the blame. In other words get other "experts" involved. There's a lot lower chance of litigation if multiple consultants have touched a case that's going into the toilet. If it does wind up in court, several others may be in line in front of you.

I also see a 3-year-old white female with a half-day of cough, congestion, body aches, and fever. The fever responds to Motrin. The child is in absolutely no distress. Here also, influenza is a possibility and we'll check for it. There are several medical options specific to influenza (depending on age): Relenza, Tambiflu, Flumadine, and Amantadine. These are antiviral medicines that can cut a couple of days off the active virus (though at significant cost and with a high side effect rate) if started within the first day or so. A flu vaccination is a better option, and surprise, the patient hasn't received one. We'll see…

Next is a 48-year-old white male with right flank pain. He was in a couple of days ago with the same symptoms. An IVP was done at that time (this is an intravenous dye study that highlights the urinary tract from the kidneys to the bladder). It was consistent with a passed stone. This morning the patient presents with a sudden onset of sharp flank pain in pretty much the same location. So, if it walks like a duck and quacks like a duck…We do another IVP to see if he's got another stone. We also give him some IV Toradol (an anti-inflammatory) and some IV fluids to try and calm things down.

I see a 33-year-old white male with pain, redness, and warmth on the dorsum (top) of his right foot. There is no history of any trauma. You at least have to think of gout (uric acid that crystallizes in the tissues) as we did in the patient earlier in the day, but the location is all wrong. New onset gout usually occurs in the first joint of the big toe. In this case, a cellulitis (a local skin infection) is more likely. There is a break in the skin at the site, and all the other findings consistent with a skin infection. These tend to be caused by bacteria from the surface of our skin (usually strep or staph) that get a foothold through a break in the skin. They then overwhelm the immune system locally. I put him on Keflex (an antibiotic with good coverage for skin organism), and Naproxen (an anti-inflammatory). The Naproxen lets me hedge my bet in case this turns out to be gout.

I see a 71-year-old white female who's congested and just can't breath very well. She's essentially got a stuffy nose and wants to be on an antibiotic. A breathing treatment doesn't do much. Given her age, I get a chest x-ray for good measure…

Our 3-year-old has a negative influenza screen. She's got a viral upper respiratory infection. There have been several of these making the rounds in the schools and daycare facilities around the area. You treat it symptomatically. I put her on Rondec DM (a cold symptom medicine), and recommend continued Tylenol or Motrin.

A squad encodes with an eighty something year old guy with a possible CVA (cerebral vascular accident or stroke). They're just minutes out.

Nursing has also triaged a 39-year-old white male to Radiology who slipped on the ice and twisted his right ankle. We'll see what it shows…

Our 21-year-old white female with low abdominal pain is back from CT. She had some vomiting just prior to going down and received some Compazine (an anti-nausea medicine) for it. Between that and the Demerol, she's feeling a bit better. We should get the CT report from the radiologist pretty shortly.

Meanwhile there's a 22-year-old white female with cough, congestion, and rib pain for the last several days. She works at UNEM (unemployed) and normally sees doctor NONE. She's essentially got a bad cold. She also would be well advised to stop smoking, but that's unlikely to happen. I give her a cold pack (antibiotic, antihistamine, and cough medicine) and send her on her way. This seems to meet her expectations.

Our 71-year-old white female with the stuffy nose has given us something of a surprise. She has pulmonary edema and is in congestive heart failure. I guess it's a good thing I got that x-ray after all. This is when she tells me that she's been having increasing leg swelling, and her weight's been climbing. She's had some recent medicine changes that she blamed. However, this is new. She's had no prior heart problems. I expand her work-up to include a complete cardiac profile. I put her on oxygen, give her an aspirin, and give her some Lasix (a diuretic). She's gone from being a person with a stuffy nose that can be managed at home, to a person who needs to be hospitalized and evaluated.

Congestive heart failure is a common, though imprecise term. It usually means that, due to some underlying cardiac pathology, the heart is unable to keep up with the demand placed upon it. In the case of left heart failure, you wind up with congestion upstream that, in this case, means fluid in the lungs. Simplistically, you get increased vascular pressures within the lungs, tissue fluids leak through into the alveoli (air sacs), and the final result is pulmonary edema (fluid in the lungs). This can be treated in a couple of ways. You can either try to make the pump work better, or you can reduce the work it needs to do. In this case, we temporarily poison the kidney's tubules with a diuretic (a water medicine) so that more urine is produced, and the load on her heart is reduced.

The real question is, "why did this happen?" This usually means that the heart is not working properly. There can be some silent coronary artery disease (hardening or narrowing of the heart's arteries), or some other type of primary heart problem. Since coronary artery disease is the most common in this age group, it is reasonable to provide cardiac protective medicines like aspirin (a blood thinner) and oxygen. She's going to need a complete cardiac work-up, and that is something I'm not going to be able to finish in the Emergency Department. I contact her doctor early, and she's admitted.

Let's not forget our 21-year-old with the abdominal pain. I finally get the radiology report, and she's apparently got a pelvic abscess. This is quite a surprise. It's no wonder she didn't get better with antibiotics, as antibiotics don't penetrate pus very well. This will need to be drained. I would be curious to know how she got this, but from my standpoint, it really doesn't matter. Her regular doctor is contacted and it becomes his problem.

12:00 PM

Oh lovely, we've got an 85-year-old code 99 inbound. This means the person has had sudden cardiac death in the field (at home), and aggressive resuscitation is in progress. The most common cause is a fatal arrhythmia, such as ventricular fibrillation or ventricular tachycardia. These are frequently in association with an acute myocardial infarction (heart attack). It sounds like the squad is 10 or 15 minutes out.

Meanwhile, I see a young 18-year-old white male with two hours of spontaneous onset one-sided testicular pain. There's no history of trauma, and he has no urinary symptoms. He has exquisite tenderness. I get him some Demerol (a strong narcotic) for pain, check a knee-jerk urinalysis, and send him off for a testicular ultrasound. These are frequently an epididymitis (an infection of the attachment to the testes, usually caused by chlamydia in an 18-year-old). However, a testicular torsion has to be ruled out.

Testicular torsion is one of the few genital emergencies in young males. They usually have a developmental defect where their testes are not properly tethered within the scrotum. Under certain circumstances the testes can twist on its stalk and shut off its blood supply. As you might imagine, this produces severe pain. If not repaired within several hours, the patient can loose the testicle.

Our squad arrives, and everything else goes on hold for a while. This is an 85-year-old white male who went down at home. It was witnessed, but we later found out that there may have been a 10 or 15 minute delay before the squad was called. The paramedics found the patient in ventricular fibrillation (where the whole heart is quivering chaotically and not pumping blood). They shocked him several times, gave several rounds of cardiac medicines, and were able to restore a stable rhythm. They intubated him in the field, and were breathing for him. Worrisome is that he is in a deep coma, and has no respiratory drive. His pupils are fixed and dilated. Given the time he was down in the field, in an 85-year-old man, there is likely irreparable brain damage. In the meantime, the patient's wife arrives. I am obligated to ask her how aggressive she wants us to be in our resuscitation. It turns out the patient did not want the types of measures that are already in play. The wife asks that we stop our support. Given the situation, this is a reasonable request. We stop our mechanical ventilation, pull the endotracheal tube, and the patient dies peacefully.

Ah well, back to the living. Our 18-year-old with the testicle pain has a normal urinalysis and an abnormal ultrasound. The on-call urologist is called, and he's taken to surgery to repair his torsion. He's someone else's problem.

Boy this is a disgusting shift. I've had essentially no time to eat or sleep, and the patients just keep on rolling in.

Next is a 35-year-old white female with a sore throat for a day. Her throat does look nasty, and the nurse has gone ahead and done a strep screen. Surprisingly, she does have a strep pharyngitis. This is the one sore throat that is treated with an antibiotic. I give her some Amoxicillin (a penicillin derivative antibiotic), some pain medicine, and send her on her way.

There are a lot of misconceptions about strep throat. It poses some risk to children, but little risk to adults. It is not the sore throat that is the issue, but the uncommon complications that can occur in the pediatric age range. The most worrisome complication is rheumatic fever and rheumatic heart disease. Antibiotics will help prevent these problems in children, but really don't significantly shorten the recovery time from the sore throat in either children or adults. It is also worth noting that not all sore throats are caused by strep, but strep throat is really the only one that responds to antibiotics. This is why the current recommendation is to only use antibiotics to treat folks with positive strep tests (at least in children).

I see a 21-year-old white male who is brought in by his wife after a witnessed seizure. He went unresponsive for several minutes and was thrashing around. By the time he reaches us he's back to baseline. He's never had anything like this happen before. I start a standard work-up, but it's unlikely we're going to find anything. The conventional wisdom of the neurologists is that everyone is entitled to one seizure. Sometimes you find the cause, but usually not. It's not until a second seizure, or if the seizure doesn't stop spontaneously, that seizure medicines are started. He has lab drawn, and is sent off for a CT scan of his head.

Meanwhile, I see a 70-year-old white male with bilateral hand swelling. Somehow he's convinced himself that a heart problem has caused his hands to swell. The biggest part of my task is to do enough to prove to him that it's not his heart. It turns out that he's being evaluated for some type of arthritis, and that a work-up is already underway to evaluate this swelling. Why he suddenly decided it was his heart, and came to my Emergency Room, I can't say. There's also a confounder that he was recently started on a medicine that has extremity swelling as a side effect. I do a full range of tests, including cardiac tests, which are normal. In the end, I have him stop his new medicine (an arthritis medicine), and put him on a taper of Prednisone (a steroid). He comments before leaving that his regular doctor had talked about putting him on cortisone (steroids). Go figure!

Our 21-year-old with the seizure is normal all down the line. He is advised to follow-up with his regular doctor the first of the week for a neurology referral.

Then I see a 30-year-old white male with right flank and back pain for a month. He had actually come in before the older gentleman who had died, but Radiology was backed up, so he was left waiting for about an hour. We have a urinalysis and a set of lumbar spine films on him that are both normal. God alone knows why he chose now to be seen for this. It's most consistent with musculoskeletal back pain. He's not really tried anything for it. I put him on my standard back regimen and suggest he follow-up if he doesn't improve.

Back pain is a common complaint in the Emergency Department. The bulk of it tends to be soft tissue injury and muscle sprains. Occasionally there are threatening causes for back pain. Sometimes these folks are drug seekers. I have adopted a systematic approach for evaluation and treatment. After a basic exam and appropriate studies, I usually put the patient of three separate medicines: an anti-inflammatory, an anti-spasmodic, and a pain medicine. The idea is to first reduce the pain with the pain pill, reduce the muscle spasm with the anti-spasmodic, and to then address the underlying inflammatory process with the anti-inflammatory. I usually run this for about 10 days. If they are no better, then a couple weeks of physical therapy is in order. Fail this, and then it might be time for a MRI. Keep in mind though, that if you do a MRI, you're really looking for something to fix surgically. I don't know about you, but I'd rather avoid someone cutting on my back at all costs. Now, of course, if there is something that suggests a significant problem right up front, then a MRI or CT might be the first test to consider, but this is really uncommon.

Heee's back! Our 25-year-old white male with the "migraine headache" that we saw early this morning is back. It seems he was okay for a couple of hours, but then his headache returned. There's some mumbling about Demerol (a strong narcotic). Not! I decide to hold onto him until we have him all-better. I would rather CT scan a person's head, or do a spinal tap on them to evaluate their headache, than give them a narcotic. I repeat the medicines he received this morning without much improvement. Then as a second pass, I give him Toradol (an injected anti-inflammatory) and Thorazine (an anti-psychotic that sometimes works with vascular headaches). Surprisingly he is completely cured. I send him out with some of the newer oral migraine medicines, and he goes away happy.

Next is a 55-year-old white male with a frontal headache for a month. This patient is a bit more worrisome, because it's like the lights are on, but nobody's home. I send him off directly to get a scan of his head.

Meanwhile I see a 74-year-old white female with increased cough and shortness of breath. Wouldn't you know it, she's a two pack a day smoker. Do you see a recurrent theme here? She gets a chest x-ray that's normal. Her symptoms are improved with a breathing treatment. She's put on some breathing medicines and an antibiotic. It's recommended that she quit smoking, and follow-up as needed. Now what's the likelihood that she's going to quit smoking? Not!

Our 55-year-old with the headache and the glassy stare has a big mother of a brain tumor. It really looks bad. There's lots of surrounding edema and it's completely distorting the architecture of the brain. He's given a big slug of steroid to try and start reducing the swelling and arrangements are made to ship him to the closest neurosurgeon. It doesn't look good. Twenty minutes later he is in a squad and headed down the road.

Okay, back to the worried well. Next in line we have a 27-year-old white male with a cough and congestion for the last few days. He's also a smoker. These repeating themes are just downright boring. Everything's normal. He gets the cold pack and is sent along.

A 30-year-old white female follows this. She's from one of the local grocery stores. She cut her finger on a meat slicer there at work. It's a very superficial flap that is pretty well deprived of any blood supply it might have had. All that can really be done for this is to dress it and let it heal on its own.

Then there's a 12-year-old white male who struck his head on a piece of concrete and sustained a scalp laceration. It's very superficial. It's cleaned and dressed. He gets head injury instructions, wound instructions, and is sent on his way.

A 2-year-old Hispanic male with clear nasal drainage, congestion and ear pain follows this. He's got a cold of course. He's also got a bilateral ear infection, so he's put on Amoxicillin (a penicillin derivative) and some cold medicines. It's recommended that he be seen again in 7-10 days to make sure the ear infection has resolved.

We have a 98-year-old white female with wrist pain since a fall two days ago. The films are fine, but she's got a nasty bruise. It'll get better.

There's a 5-year-old white male with fever and cough. He's got a cold, and is treated symptomatically.

There's a 45-year-old white male with a leg that's red from scratching. He's convinced it's infected and want's an antibiotic. I take the path of least resistance.

There's a 16-month-old white female with a cough for a day. She's had a cough off and on for months, and the parents are tired of it. Well get over it! Kids get frequent viral respiratory illnesses through the winter, and that's a fact of life! The kid has a cold.

There's a 7-year old white female with a sore throat and ear pain for two days. Her strep test is negative and her ears are fine. She's got a virus. Deal with it!

Oh joy, oh joy. We have a 28-year-old black male who's a frequent visitor. He has a range of pain complaints, and is always trying to get Demerol. He's hurt his foot, and is "sure" it's broken. Of course there is no mechanism that would break his foot, and his x-ray is normal. He then tells me that his foot pain has triggered a "migraine," and he needs something for that. And, oh yes, nothing works but Demerol. I give him some Naproxen (an anti-inflammatory) and politely tell him, in politically correct terms, "don't go away mad, just go away."

We've got a 1-year-old white male with a fever. He's got an ear infection and is put on Amoxicillin.

A 50-year-old white female with fibromyalgia follows this. She's a range of vague symptoms, and is sure she's having an allergic reaction to an antibiotic she's taking.

Fibromyalgia is a chronic pain syndrome characterized by painful trigger points. In my experience with the folks I see in the Emergency

Room, they usually have a huge psychiatric component to their illness. This lady is no exception.

In this case, I can't see any evidence that this lady is having an allergic reaction, but the path of least resistance is to treat her like she is, so I give her a shot of some antihistamine and steroid. She's happy with this and goes away a satisfied customer. This is McMedicine at its finest.

Then I've got an easy one. It's a 1-year-old Hispanic female whose mom pulled her by the arm, and now the kid doesn't want to use the arm.

This is a common injury with this mechanism. The head of the radius, in the elbow, dislocates and produces pain. It's known as "Nursemaids Elbow." It happens frequently, and is a snap to fix. You just turn the palm up, flex the elbow with one swift movement, and it pops back in.

For this patient, I do the maneuver. It's a save!

The last patient of my shift is a pregnant adolescent with a urinary tract infection, but the relief crew is here and takes over. Thank God…

I still wind up spending over an hour getting caught up on my dictation. Then I'm out of here. And not a moment too soon!

6:00 PM

Shift 2

"Fleas, ticks, and lice..."

Monday—18 Hours

12:00 PM

It sounds like things were hopping all night long. I've been off for the last 18 hours, and now, reluctantly, wade back into the fray. One of our group has been on vacation, so there have been just two of use passing off back and forth every 18 hours. The rooms are all full, but the prior shift's doc has managed to finish all those he had in progress. I guess it's time that I figuratively roll up my sleeves and get to it.

Well, let's get started. My first case is a 14-month-old white male with a welfare mom who hasn't got a clue. She's hardly more than a kid herself. Her child has a runny nose and a diaper rash. She doesn't know if he's had a fever. She doesn't have a 99¢ thermometer. However, she states that he, "seemed red" from time to time over the last day. This kid has a cold and a diaper rash. There's no emergency to speak of, and it could have easily waited until the doctor offices were open in the morning. I give the child some Rondec DM (an antihistamine/decongestant/cough medicine) for the cold symptoms and some Lotrimin (an antifungal cream) for the diaper rash. I really need the ability to prescribe parenting classes for the mom (or a contraceptive before the fact).

Something we frequently talk about is how folks need to pass a test and get a license to do something as basic as drive a care, but that anyone can have a kid. If you think about it, bringing a child into the world and indoctrinating it into a life of welfare and poverty has a much greater social impact than just about anything else a person can do.

I see way too many children 11, 12, 13, 14, and 15 having children themselves. Hell, one is too many! In some parts of the local black community it almost seems like a right of passage for these young girls to have their first child by age 15 or so. They make statements like, "my mom had me when she was 14!" as though it is a justification and validation of the act of adolescent pregnancy. I'm not being racist here, this is just my experience.

I think youth pregnancy is a real problem in our society that we are unrealistic about solving. "Just abstain!" is not a practical answer. The assertion that sex education should take place at home is hopelessly naive; the reality is that it just isn't happening. I see this as such a large societal problem that it should be handled systematically. I think that sex education and birth control should be taught from the time children are capable of understanding the issues. I think that reality-based child rearing and responsibility training should occur in step with this. This would de-glamorize having babies to this youthful set, and introduce them to the fact that children are a 24 hour a day, 7 day a week, lifetime project. I also believe that there should be more research on effective birth control options, and that birth control should be both universally available and free to all. Well, so much for my soapbox! I see the tragedy of not facing these issues in my Emergency Room every day, and so much of it could be prevented.

Back to the task at hand. The next patient is a 64-year-old white female who twisted her left knee when she tripped over the family pet. She's got severe knee pain and is having a hard time bearing weight. Her x-rays show an unusual fracture of the tibial spines (small bony prominences inside the knee). This is usually associated with injury to the big ligaments in the knee, the cruciates. I talk it over with the local orthopedic surgeon. Then I put her in a knee immobilizer, give her some symptomatic medicines, and refer her to the orthopedic doctor of her choice for follow-up.

A 60-year-old white female with a red mattery eye and a cough follows this. Her grandchild had an eye infection earlier in the week, and she thinks she may have picked it up from her. Except for her eye, there aren't many findings on exam. I put her on some antibiotic eye drops and some symptomatic medicines for her cough.

I also see a 27-year-old white male with headache for a day. He states that he gets them weekly these days, and that this is more frequent than normal. Otherwise it is his usual headache. His exam is normal. I give him routine headache medicines, and wait to see how he does.

Next is a 26-year-old obese white male who slipped on ice yesterday. He fell backwards striking the back of his head. He had a few seconds of loss of consciousness. He was seen at a nearby medical facility, a CT of his head was done, and it was normal. He presents today because he has a persistent posterior headache with nausea. He and his family are convinced that he has some severe brain injury. His exam is normal. This is likely a benign post-concussion syndrome, but the family is obligating me to repeat his head scan. I send him off to Radiology, knowing it's going to be another normal scan.

Meanwhile I see a 35-year-old white male who has had neck pain for several weeks. It began when he was rear-ended at a stop sign. He had seen his regular doctor and had some films of his neck done. They were normal. He's just been on pain pills off and on, and has not bothered to follow-up further with his regular doctor. So of course, it's an emergency today. This is managed pretty much the same way I handle acute back pain. After a normal exam, I put him on all the right medicines.

I then see a 70-year-old obese white male with right hip pain for several hours. He has no history of any specific trauma. He is triaged to Radiology for good measure. His films are, of course, normal except for expected arthritic change. His pain begins at a point in his buttocks where the sciatic nerve comes close to the surface. This fellow was a truck driver for most of his working life, and had just taken a cross-country trip. It looks like he's flared up this nerve, and has himself a case of sciatica. He's put on an anti-inflammatory and some pain medicine. He can follow-up as needed.

Our 26-year-old is back from CT, and surprise, it's another normal scan! He and his family are provided reassurance. His symptoms are better with just some Tylenol. He's given routine head injury instructions and sent on his way.

Now it's time for a trio of dueling 90-year-olds...

First I see a 90-year-old white female with a three-day history of increasing shortness of breath. She smokes like a chimney, and has done so all her life. She's huffing and puffing to beat the band. Her oxygen saturation is in the low 80% range on room air. Multiple breathing treatments and 6 liters per minute of oxygen by nasal cannula, and she's just barely into the 90% saturation range (normal is usually 95-100%). Her chest x-ray shows a little bit of heart failure, but not enough to account for all of the symptoms. She's given some Lasix (a diuretic) to mobilize some of the fluid. Several studies are initiated, but she's a keeper. With her long smoking history she probably has some baseline lung disease. Her symptoms are probably what we know as exacerbation of COPD (chronic obstructive lung disease). This is stressing her heart enough to give her a bit of heart failure as well. I'm not going to be able to figure it all out down here, so I contact her doctor, and we get her admitted.

Second of our trio is a 90-year-old white female with a red, swollen, hot, tender ankle that she noticed this morning. There's no history of trauma, and no systemic signs or symptoms. She has a localized cellulitis, a bacterial infection involving her ankle. This is usually skin bacteria that gets a foothold on the underlying tissue. It usually responds quickly to an oral antibiotic if caught early. This patient is allergic to penicillins, and so I put her on Keflex (an inexpensive antibiotic with good coverage for skin infections) instead. It is noteworthy that there is a 10% crossover allergy with this antibiotic for folks who are allergic to penicillin, so I warn her to keep an eye out for possible side effects.

Last in our trio is a 90-year-old white female with recurrent chest pain for the last several days. She has a significant cardiac history including a three-vessel heart bypass ten or twelve years before. She's been having this pain both with exertion and at rest. It lasts for up to an hour at a time. When it occurs, it radiates to her back, and has associated severe shortness of breath. She's just convinced its indigestion. NOT! She has new EKG changes as well as new pulmonary edema (fluid in her lungs) on her chest x-ray. She's having no active symptoms at presentation.

Now is as good a time as any to say a few words about the management of cardiac chest pain. Well what do you do about it all?

When a person comes in with chest pain there is an initial EKG and a review of their history and risk factors. It isn't always completely clear from their history whether chest pain is cardiac or not. The goal is to try and decipher this and to minimize risk of a bad outcome regardless.

If there is a strong suspicion that a patient is having angina or unstable angina (heart pain), then there are several protective things that are done that have been shown to decrease risk of progression to infarction (heart attack) and associated injury of the heart muscle. A patient is usually given an aspirin; this acts as a blood thinner and reduces risk of spontaneous small blood clots that can precipitate a heart attack in a person with narrowed heart vessels. They are put on oxygen to maximize oxygen delivery to the heart. They are given nitroglycerine, which dilates blood vessels to improve coronary artery flow and reduce arterial spasm. They are given beta-blockers (Lopressor, Tenormin) that decrease the load on the heart by slowing it, thereby reducing the effect of stress hormones by blocking their receptors. Finally, they are given a heparin-like compound (Heparin, Lovenox), which further acts to thin their blood and reduce risk of clot formation. Some or all of these interventions frequently produce a complete resolution of pain.

If a person is actually having a heart attack, the preceding is done, but in addition they are evaluated for TPA (tissue plasminogen activator, the clot busting drug). They may also need some morphine to help with pain and anxiety. These actions are usually enough to deal with the immediate risks in an acute heart attack. Rarely, they are inadequate, and in that case, the patient gets referred for emergent angioplasty (the balloon). My facility does not have this ability, and so these patients are shipped to a larger nearby hospital that offers these services. Sometimes in these larger hospitals, angioplasty occurs in lieu of TPA, just because you can kill two birds with one stone. You can both evaluate the coronary arteries, and open any blockages that you find by dilating the stenotic arteries. In addition, stents are sometimes used to prop open these newly dilated vessels. These are tubular wire mesh devices that are opened in the previously narrowed area. They act to shore up the vessel walls until the body is able to take care of that task on its own.

Now our 90-year-old is already on aspirin and a beta-blocker. She is put on some oxygen, some nitroglycerine paste, some Lovenox (heart protective medicines), and some additional Lasix (a diuretic). Her regular doctor is contacted in short order, she is out of here!

I know it may not appear that I'm doing much work, but to me it seems like I no sooner finish one patient than the next one shows up. It's not quit as bad as the last shift (not so much death and destruction), but it's only slightly better.

All right then, let's get back to the worried well. I see a 39-year-old white female with cough, congestion, and sinus drainage for about a week. Of course she's a pack a day smoker and not motivated to quit. She's got some sinus pressure as well, so probably has a sinusitis. She gets a cold pack and is sent on her way.

I get an 8-year-old white male who was playing baseball in the house and ran into the wall. He split his forehead open. He needs half a dozen stitches. You'd swear we were killing him, given the fuss he puts up.

Then I see a real winner. It's a 70-year-old white male with a cough and sore throat for a month. It's a crisis today. Apparently the sore throat is worse. Now you always have to ask, with chronic symptoms like this in an older man, if there could perhaps be a laryngeal malignancy involved. I'm not going to find this out in the Emergency Room. He needs follow-up, and a day one way or the other isn't going to make any difference. He wants an antibiotic, so I give him one. I also give him something for the discomfort. He is told to follow-up.

Later we get an 18-year-old white female who twisted her ankle in a fall on the ice. She's incredibly dramatic. Of course, her x-rays are normal. She gets routine sprain treatment. She's put in an air splint, put on crutches, and can follow-up as needed.

There's a 18-year-old white female who dropped a dish in the kitchen and cut her leg. I yuck it up with her while I get her leg put back together. It takes a handful of stitches, and she's sent on her way.

A 6-year-old white female with a one-day history of sore throat and left ear pain follows this. Her ear is fine, but she does have strep throat. Frequently, with sore throats there is often enough inflammation in the back of the throat that the eustachian tubes become dysfunctional. The eustachian tubes act to equalize the atmospheric pressure behind the eardrums. It's like what happens if you ride on an airplane when you've got a sinus infection, your ears hurt. She's put on some Amoxicillin (a penicillin based antibiotic) and given some symptomatic medicines.

Finally, there's a 46-year-old white female with a cough, body aches, and shortness of breath for a day. Of course she's also smoker, about 2 packs a day. She also has a history of asthma. Interesting combination, don't you think? Sometimes I think people are their own worst enemy. She gets a whole lot better with a breathing treatment. I do a chest x-ray and get an influenza screen for good measure. They're normal. She's put on a cold pack plus an inhaler. I try to impress on her that the bulk of her symptoms are due to her smoking, but she doesn't want to hear it. Ah, well…

Well, now it's time for something I can look forward to, dinner! I didn't have the opportunity to have lunch, so I'm starving. The cafeteria food is underwhelming, but I manage just the same.

6:00 PM

Well, there's a slight reprieve from the unwashed masses. I use this to get caught up on my dictation. This only lasts for about an hour, and we're back and running…

A 60-year-old white male who had what we term a "spell" at the dinner table interrupts my lament. He was sitting at the table, stared off into space for a while, during which he didn't respond, and then returned to baseline. He'd had a similar episode a few months ago, and had a huge work-up at the time without any real specific findings. I do my standard syncope work-up, although this really isn't true syncope. I don't hit on anything except for the fact that the guy's three sheets to the wind. His blood alcohol is just about three times the legal limit. In talking more with the wife, it sounds like he's been having these spells for some time. Occasionally, he has some twitching. It sounds like he's even had a couple of full-blown grand mal seizures. He's probably just having alcohol-associated seizures. It's all part of what I refer to as "pickled brain syndrome." He's been drinking a long time, and is unlikely to stop anytime soon, so he's going to have to live with it. He can talk to his regular doctor about a seizure medicine, but it's hard to tell how effective it would be. It's also really questionable whether he would be compliant with taking it.

A lot of people don't realize just how common alcoholism is in the elderly. I see folks all the time, even in their 80's and 90's, who come in dead drunk. Usually it's the case of young drunks aging into old drunks, but not always. Interesting thought, huh?

Next is an 8-month-old hispanic female with nausea, vomiting, and diarrhea for a day. She's happy as a clam, but the mother insists through the interpreter that she just vomits up everything she is given. Of course, the mother keeps trying to feed her formula every time she vomits, and so it isn't real rocket science that the child is likely to vomit. She doesn't seem to know the basics of dealing with a vomiting child. I give the child a Phenergan suppository (an anti-nausea medicine) for good measure, wait a while, and let her try some Pedialyte (a rehydration solution available in any grocery store). It stays down, the kid stays happy, the mom's happy, everyone's happy. She likely has the stomach bug that's been making the rounds. A couple weeks ago I was seeing 8-12 people a shift with this. With most folks it's been a 24-hour bug.

Then I see a 2-year-old hispanic male, a two-fer in the same room as the 8-month-old. He's been fussy and has a cough. He does have a red eardrum, and so has an ear infection in addition to his cold. I put him on some Amoxicillin (a penicillin derivative antibiotic), and some symptomatic medicines. He needs his ear rechecked in a week or so.

Hmmm, we're starting to have a trend here. Next is a 2-year-old white female with right ear pain and vomiting. She also has a red eardrum. So she has an ear infection in addition to a stomach bug. Everything else is normal. I give her a shot of Rocephin (a broad-spectrum antibiotic with a 95% single-dose effectiveness for ear infection). Otherwise she gets routine vomiting instructions. She too needs to be rechecked in a week or so.

Then we get a "real" emergency, a three-fer with head lice. It's a 4, 6, and 8-year-old set of siblings brought in with the little critters. The parents act like their children are dying because of these insects, and want something done "right away." I mention to them that pretty much all of the lice preparations on the market are available over-the-counter. Well the long and the short of it is that these folks are on Medicaid. If they can get a prescription, then they don't have to pay for it themselves. Fine, whatever! I guess you and I will buy it for them.

Next, we have a repeat of earlier in the shift. It's a 28-year-old white female who yesterday had fallen and struck the back of her head. Tonight she feels nauseated and is sure she has some dire brain injury. So, of course, I'm pretty much obligated to scan her brain and prove that she's going to live to see another day. And guess what? It's normal! Surprise, surprise.

A 28-year-old white female who twisted her foot and has pain across the top of her foot follows this. It's filmed. It's normal. She's treated and streeted.

Sometimes I feel like I should have gone to dental school as well as medical school given the number of folks who come to the ER for their dental problems. I see a 23-year-old white female with tooth pain for four months. I guess its worse tonight. She hasn't wanted to have it taken care of when it was an inexpensive problem, and instead chooses now to come and visit me. It doesn't seem to matter that the cost of this one ER visit would probably pay for a year of dental care for this girl. All I'm going to do is temporize it. She's got a cavity that involves half her second molar on the bottom, and given what's draining from it, it's infected to boot. I put her on an antibiotic and give her something for pain. I try and impress on her that she really does need to see a dentist, if only to have the tooth pulled. From the looks of things, she's likely to start having problems with her wisdom teeth here pretty soon as well.

The witching hour is approaching and wouldn't you know it, the crazy people are out in force. This is in the form of a 62-year-old white male who presents because he has a dry mouth and feels tingly all over. He's just sure he's having a heart attack. He's has no chest pain, nor is he short of breath. He's very active, and regularly uses his treadmill without any problem. He just strikes me as the nervous, anxious type. Of course his EKG is completely normal. The second Xanax (a fast acting tranquilizer) cures him. I give him a supply of Xanax to last him until he can see his regular doctor, and send him on out the door.

12:00 AM

Here's something I don't see very often. It's a 30-year-old white female who's about 12 weeks pregnant, and hasn't been able to pee for the last 12 hours. She's pretty uncomfortable. This usually means they have a urinary tract infection, but her urinalysis was normal. A bladder scan (a special ultrasound to measure the amount of urine in the bladder) is done that shows well over a quart of urine in her bladder.

She gets a foley catheter (a tube in her bladder), and feels much better when her bladder is drained. The catheter is left in place. She can follow-up with her regular doctor later in the morning.

This lady's problem is likely due to the pregnant uterus flopping down against the bladder outlet. As the fetus enlarges and lifts the uterus out of the pelvis, this is going to correct itself.

A 24-year-old white female with a 20-minute history of sharp left-sided chest pain follows this. It's worse with movement and a deep breath. She's convinced she's having a heart attack. Not! The probability of someone her age having a heart attack is essentially zero. She has asthma and is a smoker. She gets a breathing treatment and a chest x-ray. She's essentially got pleurisy, an inflammation of the lining of the lung that is more common in smokers. I give her some symptomatic medicines and send her on her way. She's still not convinced that she's not having a heart attack. Ah well, win some, loose some.

I hear my pillow calling. My dictation can wait...

Zzzz...

3:00 AM

Well so much for sleeping! The huddled masses are upon me. There's an 80-year-old white male who hasn't been able to pee for the last 6-8 hours and is feeling uncomfortable. He has a known prostate cancer that's getting irradiated. Because of this, he has chronic blood in his urine. We drop a foley catheter into his bladder, and drain a quart of bloody urine. The urinalysis suggests it may be infected as well. I put him on Levaquin (an antibiotic). I leave the catheter in place, and will let him follow-up later in the morning with his urologist.

A 55-year-old white male with a severe one-sided sore throat follows this. It doesn't help that he's a nut as well, so he's got a million other complaints. Most concerning is that he does have quite a bit more throat swelling on the one side. A peritonsillar abscess becomes a possibility. This is a collection of pus under the tonsil that can be threatening if not drained. I check some lab for good measure, but then arrange for him the get a CT scan of his neck. It takes forever to get the CT tech in to do the scan.

Meanwhile, I see a 3-year-old white female with a fever and "breathing problems." I'm sorry, but the kid has a cold. The parents are older, first time, parents. I get the impression that the child is taken to the doctor for every little thing. I wind up having to submit her to a range of indignities in order to convince the parents that she's fine. Sometimes I just have to shake my head.

Well so much for sleeping…

The scan on our 55-year-old is fine. The strep test is positive. He gets an antibiotic, something for pain, and can follow-up as needed.

5:30 AM

I jokingly comment, "where's our morning chest pain?" It was a three day weekend, and this is the equivalent of a Monday morning. Statistically, there are more heart attacks and chest pain cases on Monday mornings, or whatever day is the first day of work for the week. I swear, not fifteen minutes from the statement, a chest pain rolls in.

It's a 70-year-jold white male with two hours of chest pain and shortness of breath. Within the last week he had had a heart catheterization and was found to have a 90% blockage in one vessel. It was angioplastied and stented.

A relatively common complication with angioplasty is what is known as early reocclusion. The freshly dilated heart artery does not have a normal endothelium, the inner lining. Clot can form at this area and block the recently opened artery. Sometimes these folks need repeat angioplasty to open it back up.

Some nitrates and oxygen, and this gentleman is symptom free. Of course he gets all of the other protective medicines as well. I call his regular doctor and he is admitted right away. I anticipate that they will probably ship him off to the cath lab and repeat his heart catheterization to make sure their handy work is still doing what it should.

Regardless, he's out of my department, my relief is here, and so I am out of here....

I've actually got a few days off. I've got to finish the final proofs on my last book, as well as get all of this typed up. Oh joy.

6:00 AM

Shift 3

"If you hear hoof beats don't look for zebras...Ah, most of the time..."

Saturday—18 Hours

6:00 AM

It's hard to believe I've been off for a whole four days. It took one full day to recover from the long weekend, two days to transcribe my adventures, and that left me with essentially one day off to do other stuff. The weather has been warmer, and the snow is starting to melt. It still refreezes every night, and makes driving and walking quite a challenge. I commute about 60 miles to work, so weather and road conditions can be very significant issues.

As I walk through the door, the scene looks grim. Outside, the parking lot is completely full. There are squads and police units idling nearby, and this is an ominous sign. The lobby is completely full and more folks appear to be wandering in. My first impulse is to turn around and go the other way. My over-riding moniker for the Emergency Department is that, "boredom is a good thing!" And this does not look like boredom. Lots of excitement means more potential to make mistakes, and increased likelihood of facing litigation. An ideal shift for me is one where I go the whole stretch without seeing a single patient. This is euphemistically known as, "sleeping for dollars." There's not much chance of that these days. One thing I've really noticed about emergency medicine in the last five years it that the volumes of folks using the Emergency Department as their primary source of medical care has risen dramatically. This is not a good sign.

The doc I'm relieving looks like he's VERY happy to see me. Every room is full, and there is complete and utter chaos. This does not bode well for an early Saturday morning. Local doctor's offices are typically open until noon on Saturday, so we usually don't see this level of activity until well into the afternoon.

My first task of the morning is to assume the care of a 50-year-old white male who has had chest pressure and slight shortness of breath since the previous evening. He has also been having nausea, vomiting, and diarrhea. He points to his upper mid-abdomen as the point where he has most of his discomfort. He thought it was indigestion or a stomach bug, but it isn't getting any better. He's been a smoker since he was a teen, and has been told his cholesterol is "a little high." His EKG has some subtle changes, but there is nothing definitive. There are no old EKGs to compare with to see if these changes are old or new. The patient has no significant past medical history to speak of. My initial impression is that this is probably non-cardiac, but I've been fooled before, so I tend to maintain a very high index of suspicion. I start a routine cardiac work-up, and try some maneuvers to see if I can improve upon his discomfort.

Emergency Departments are pretty consistent in how they handle chest pain. Since cardiac chest pain is something where you are potentially racing against the clock in order to reduce risk of permanent disability and death, folks with chest pain are typically immediately triaged into the department for evaluation. Rule of thumb goals are to have an EKG done and interpreted within 20 minutes, and TPA (the clot buster drug) running (where appropriate) within an hour of hitting the door. Though this sounds straight forward, it's not always as easy as all that.

A routine Emergency Department cardiac work-up typically includes a range of things. An EKG is done as mentioned, and sometimes more that one are required over time. In addition, there is lab done which includes a blood count, basic electrolytes, heart enzyme levels (creatinine kinase and troponin), and coagulation factors. A portable chest x-ray is usually done as well. Of course, all this doesn't occur immediately, but usually takes about an hour or so. Sometimes it can take quite a bit longer, if the lab is really busy.

It is worth nothing that not all chest pain is cardiac in origin. In fact, depending on demographics, risk factors, and the like, the probability of cardiac chest pain can range from essentially zero to 100%. The obvious cardiac chest pain is usually very apparent, and there's no question. The really tuff ones are the atypical chest pain. This later group is often the bulk of patients presenting to the Emergency Department. The downside of public chest pain awareness programs is that it prompts everyone, young and old, low risk and high risk, to come to the ER at the first twinge of chest discomfort. It's not practical or economic to do a full cardiac evaluation on every one of these that shows up, so the ER physician has to weigh the relative risk factors in each case. Since missed heart attack is one of the highest malpractice judgments out there, the stakes are very high to always get it right.

Well back to our 50-year-old. He's given an aspirin and put on some oxygen. An IV is started, and he's given some sublingual nitroglycerine (a medicine that dilates heart vessels and helps cardiac chest pain). The nitro doesn't really help. The patient has a history of ulcer disease, so a rectal exam is done to make sure he's not bleeding into his gut. He's not. He's given other heart protective medicines more as a knee-jerk. The thought is that we've done good if it turns out to be cardiac, and have really done no harm if it doesn't. This includes a heart slowing medicine, Lopressor, and a blood thinner, Lovenox. None of them really helps his ongoing pain, so we hang a nitroglycerine drip, and start titrating some Morphine (a narcotic pain medicine) as well. The lab is cooking. We'll just keep pressing forward.

In the meantime, I see a 28-year-old white female with an alleged "migraine headache" for the last two hours. She tells me that nothing works but Demerol (a strong narcotic). NOT! This is a perfectly healthy appearing young woman who is classified as disabled. She has no apparent disability that I can ascertain.

I really wonder who signs off on these disability issues? I see a huge number of able-bodied people who are unemployed or who are allegedly disabled. I just don't understand it.

I explain to this patient that I'm not going to be giving her Demerol. She's not happy with this, and she then tries to negotiate for her other narcotics of choice. This negotiation continues throughout her stay, both directly and through the nurse. She finally settles for a few Talwin NX (a non-narcotic pain medicine) and goes away. I just get so frustrated with the narcotic and prescription medicine seekers. These folks are often the most ardent complainers and letter writers to administration, and I'm constantly getting raked over the coals about their complaints. Hence back to my McMedicine analogy. I'll do what I can to keep all these idiots happy, but there are some lines I will not cross. If they don't like it, well tough!

Then back to our 50-year-old. He's got unmistakable cardiac enzyme elevations consistent with a recent or ongoing heart attack. He's also sucking up enough Morphine to render a small elephant unconscious, with little impact on his pain. I don't have strong enough criteria to give TPA (there are specific criteria that must be met to ensure the benefits of the drug outweigh the risks). This guy really needs an emergent heart catheterization. I contact the on-call cardiologist but he hems and haws about it. None-the-less I put a helicopter on stand-by. The closest cath lab is in the next city over.

I then pop in and see a little 6-year-old white male, patient of doctor NONE, who has had a fever, sore throat, nausea and vomiting. The nurse has gone ahead and gotten a strep screen, and it was positive. The kid has strep throat. I get him a shot of long acting penicillin, as well as some nausea meds, and send him on his way. He'll be fine.

I finally get the go-ahead from the cardiologist. I call in the chopper, and my 50-year-old flies off to get his heart arteries explored.

Next is a 39-year-old white female who works at UNEM (unemployed). She's had hip pain for a week. There's no history of trauma, and she's been taking nothing for her pain. A therapeutic x-ray is done, because the patient expects it, and it shows some degenerative change. She's perhaps 150 pounds overweight, which is likely the source of her hip pain. I put her on an anti-inflammatory and send her on her way.

A 35-year-old white female follows this, with a painful breast for the last several days. There's some redness, swelling, and tenderness. It looks like mastitis (a bacterial infection of the glandular tissue of the breast that is more common in women who are breast-feeding). This woman isn't breastfeeding. I put her on dicloxacillin (an appropriate antibiotic) and give her something for discomfort. I insist that she follow-up. There are some rare forms of breast cancer that can present this way. It needs to be explored further if it doesn't rapidly clear up.

I also see a 26-year-old white female with three days of back pain. There is no history of trauma. She's very dramatic. She's been seeing a chiropractor, and her pain is worse. Her exam is pretty normal. I do some therapeutic x-rays and put her on my routine back pain regimen.

This is a pretty good place to do my little diatribe on chiropractors. They can really do well for a patient if they stick to those areas where research has shown that they excel. Chiropractors do very well with many folks with chronic low back pain. Unfortunately, there seem to be a lot of unscrupulous practitioners out there who make claims that they can cure everything from diabetes to cancer by "adjusting" folks backs. They also sell a wide range of expensive vitamins and supplements with very hyped claims of dubious validity. This really reflects poorly on chiropractors as a group. I also hear a lot of claims about necks and backs being "out of alignment" and how an "adjustment" restores this alignment. I defy any chiropractor to show me before and after x-rays that demonstrate a restored "alignment" after an adjustment. Ah well, so much for my rant.

A squad is encoding. It seems there is an 85-year-old white female inbound from home with weakness and confusion. She's been in a lot and keeps winding up back in the nursing home. Unfortunately, she signs herself out of the nursing home, goes back home, and fails there yet again. Ah well. It's a seemingly endless cycle.

12:00 PM

First though, I see an 18-year-old white male who has recurrent right upper abdomenal pain. He was just through the million-dollar work-up within the last couple of weeks with no specific findings. I start reinventing the wheel, repeating prior studies, to see if I can find something else that points me in the right direction. We'll see…

The Emergency Department is frequently placed in the position of being the point of service for second opinions. Folks whose regular physicians are unable to figure out what's going on, or who are not confident with what their physicians have told them, frequently wind up in the ER to get it figured out. Now sometimes we get lucky, and do manage to sort stuff out, just because we are more aggressive. But many times, especially with chronic problems that have already seen all the experts, we are woefully inadequate to the task. Most folks don't realize that the ER has only a small subset of testing available to it. We are set up to find immediately threatening conditions. Anything beyond that is a bonus.

About this time our 85-year-old weak and confused person shows up by squad. She is more confused than normal, and so I start my standard delirium work-up. This includes lab, chest x-ray, EKG, and head scan looking for reversible causes of confusion.

I also get a second squad in about the same time with another 85-year-old white female with a cough for a week. She normally gets all of her medical care in a nearby city, but comes to our ER today by squad because it's convenient. She does have an oxygen saturation that's in the seventies, but doesn't admit to being overly short of breath, except with exertion. She has a history of pneumonia, and I'll be surprised if that's not what's going on now. She's put on some oxygen and given a breathing treatment. Lab and a chest x-ray are ordered.

Meanwhile, I see a 9-year-old white female who's had right ear pain for 3 weeks. She's had some increased drainage today, so the mom decided it was time for her to be seen. She's got an infection both in the ear canal and behind the eardrum. I put her on some oral antibiotic as well as some antibiotic drops. She can follow-up. Why is it a crisis today? Who knows?

There's also a 4-year-old white male who has fallen at home while playing on a piece of furniture. He has a tiny scalp laceration. I quickly put a skin staple in it so he can be on his way.

I also see a 79-year-old white male with right hip pain for an hour. There was no trauma, and he's tried nothing for it. I send him over for a film.

Back to the 85-year-old confused lady. I'm really not finding much of anything. Then she starts having 10 of 10 chest pain. She does have known severe heart disease that is inoperable, and is likely having unstable angina. However, I wouldn't put it past her to fake it in order to be admitted to the hospital. She's done this before. She is cured with two nitroglycerine tablets. I call her regular doctor and arrange for her to be admitted.

Our other 85-year-old has a big pneumonia. She's decided she wants to stay here rather than going to see her regular doctor. Again, this is because it is convenient for her and her family. I call and make arrangements to find her a doctor. She gets queued up for admission.

By this time our 79-year-old with the hip pain is back from Radiology. He has a lot of degenerative change on the film, but otherwise nothing. I put him on an arthritis medicine and send him on his way.

A 14-year-old white male comes in complaining of right ankle pain after playing basketball, and is sent to Radiology.

Meanwhile, our 18-year-old with the belly pain is feeling all-better. His lab is normal. His belly films do have a few dilated loops of small bowel. It's about this point that I get one of those, "oh, by the way…,"

comments from the parents. It seems he's had several abdominal oper-
ations as a child. Now this is significant because the list of potential
causes of abdominal pain goes up in someone who's had a surgeon in
their belly. It makes it possible that the belly films mean this kid's
developing a bowel obstruction rather than having a stomach bug.
This kid gets passed off to the surgery folks.

Boy the patient load is just not slowing down.

Our 14-year-old has normal ankle films, and I treat it like the sprain
it is.

There's also a 15-year-old white male that the ER nurse had sent for
x-ray. He jammed his thumb. He's got a little chip fracture, is splinted,
and advised to follow-up.

Then it's time for the next squad. It's a 100-year-old white female with
a hoarse voice and cough. I get a chest x-ray for good measure (normal),
and put her on both an antibiotic and some symptomatic medicines.

As if I'm not having enough fun, the next person is a 48-year-old
white female that I would put into the category of nut. She complains
of having "too much adrenaline." She refuses to even consider that
this could be anxiety related, although she is cured with a Xanax (a
tranquilizer). She has what we euphemistically call "hypo-
Xanaxemia" (not enough antianxiety medicine). We sometimes joke
that we ought to put tranquilizers and antidepressants in the drinking
water. Maybe we'd have fewer visits from these crazies. She goes on
her way.

And we're back to the geriatric cases. It's an 80-year-old white
female with an hour of chest pain, and increasing shortness of breath
for the last few days. She's got a borderline oxygen saturation. Her
EKG is nonspecific, but her chest x-ray is one big white-out. She's got
florid pulmonary edema (fluid in the lungs). She's a keeper, so I call
her doctor early in the scheme of things and she's out of here quickly.

Then we're back to the more mundane. It's a 27-year-old white
female with a sore throat for a week. She wants an antibiotic, so I don't
even bother to see if she has strep. Why do a $50 test if you're going to

ignore the results? So fine, I give her a $10 antibiotic and send her out the door.

This is followed immediately by a 40-year-old white male who's been under treatment for bronchitis for the last week. He continues to smoke 2 packs of cigarettes a day and can't understand why he's not getting better. His chest x-ray is fine. I give him a breathing treatment, and he feels better. I arrange for him to have a nebulizer (this was his agenda from the start), and send him out. He refuses to accept that his continued smoking could have anything to do with his respiratory illness.

Then it's time for a diagnostic dilemma. It's a 55-year-old white male who comes in by squad after a day of shortness of breath. He gets all of his health care elsewhere, but is here for the convenience. He is crazy as a loon. Unfortunately, he's got aplastic anemia. His bone marrow is failing, and he requires repeat transfusions of blood and platelets to stay alive. So, despite his nuttiness, he could have almost anything going on. When it comes to folks with malignancies, testing and evaluation is always a challenge. Almost every test is abnormal. It is often difficult to tell if a test is abnormal enough to actually mean something. This patient is no exception. Pretty much every test I do is abnormal. The patient is in no distress, so I wait to collect more information before I get more aggressive.

In the meantime I see a 20-year-old white female with left flank pain off and on for the last 3 weeks. It's worse today. Of course she's not had it looked into at any time since it started. She has a history of kidney stones, and she acts like she's got one now. These folks usually act like they're sitting on hot coals. They keep moving around, and just can't get comfortable. The nurse has gotten a urinalysis that is chock full of blood. This is pretty typical of a kidney stone. I get some other lab and order an IVP (a x-ray dye study that is used to identify kidney stones). In the meantime, I have her started on some IV fluids, and give her some IV Toradol (an anti-inflammatory).

And we've got yet another squad. It's a 30-year-old white male, a real road warrior, who had a possible seizure. He's totally unresponsive. He's drunk as a skunk on alcohol, and who knows what else. He has hardly a square inch of his body that's not covered by tattoos. It's looking like he may need to be intubated to protect his airway, but then he starts waking up and doing well on his own. I do a range of tests including an alcohol level and drug screen. Initially I was going to scan his head as well, but with him waking up, I put it on hold.

Back to our guy with the aplastic anemia. He's got an EKG that's very abnormal. He could be infarcting. He has essentially no white cells (infection fighting cells) and no platelets (clotting cells). Luckily his hemoglobin is normal, so he must have had a recent transfusion. His heart enzymes are elevated, as is his D-Dimer (a measure of clot product that can suggest blood clot). His blood pressure is marginal. I have him on some oxygen, some IV fluids, and have given him some Lopressor to slow his heart down a bit. I chat with the cardiologist, but he hasn't got a real clue on how to proceed with a patient like this. The majority of the heart protective medicines could kill a person with no platelets like this guy. I call this person's oncologist, but he tells me that he has nothing to offer, that it's a cardiology problem. I decide to temporize, and order a spiral CT of this guy's chest to see if he may have a blood clot sitting in his lungs. How someone with no platelets could form a blood clot is beyond me, but my objective findings require that I investigate this option as a real possibility.

6:00 PM

And if all this isn't enough, I have to see a 44-year-old white male with a "migraine headache." He's a drug seeker from way back. I tell him right up front that he's not going to get any Demerol, and he agrees to take what I give him. I'm surprised. He's out the door quickly.

I've also got a 70-year-old white male with a history of thyroid cancer. He's had his thyroid removed months ago, and has persistent recurrent hoarseness. He's just tired of it and so decided it was time to get it evaluated in the ER. He's already been to his surgeon and his oncologist several times about this. What the hell am I supposed to do about it? I get a quick chest x-ray, offer symptomatic medicines, and refer him back to the local ENT doctor to see what he might have to say about it.

Our road warrior has a blood alcohol that's about twice the legal limit. He also tests positive for pretty much everything on our drug screen. He's awake now, and surprisingly articulate and polite. He likely had a seizure. This was perhaps triggered by some combination of his poly-substance abuse. He wants to go home with a friend. I can't think of any good reason for him not to go, and so I send him on his way.

Our 20-year-old with flank pain has a kidney stone. It looks like she's about to pass it. She was immediately pain free with the Toradol. She's given some pain pills, told to get plenty of fluids, strain her urine, and follow-up with her regular doctor.

Our 50-year-old guy with the aplastic anemia has a pulmonary embolus. There's blood clot in most of the big vessels in one lung. I talk to the local doctors, who feel he should be shipped to a higher level of care. I talk again with the guy's oncologist who states that he has nothing to offer unless there is clot in the patient's legs. If there is, then a filter could be placed in the big vessel going up to the heart to catch clot and prevent a bigger blood clot from moving to the lungs. It doesn't take much deducing to figure that this patient's regular doctor does not want him back! I order an ultrasound of his legs to see if I can get more justification to ship him to a higher level of care.

But first, I have a bit more disease and pestilence to stomp out. I see a 3-month-old white male with a low-grade fever who's fussy. The kid looks fine. He might have the start of a little ear infection. I cover him for that and send him along.

Second is a 55-year-old white female with stomach and back pain for 2 weeks. It's no better or worse tonight. I do a range of testing, but don't find anything specific. I treat her symptomatically, and suggest she follow-up.

Third is an 80-year-old white male who caught his foot on the sharp edge of a rack at home and lacerated his foot. It takes about a dozen sutures to repair.

Fourth is a 15-year-old white male who got a finger in the eye while playing basketball. He wound up with a black eye out of it, scraped the sclera (the white part) of the eye, but otherwise has no significant injury. He's given some antibiotic eye drops, something for pain, and is sent on his way.

Fifth is a 20-year-old white female with hives. She's had no specific new exposure. This is an allergic reaction to something, but we often don't find out what. I give her some steroids and an antihistamine, and she's all-better.

Sixth is the 20-year-old white female I'd seen earlier with urinary symptoms. She had a borderline urinalysis then. Now she's had a single episode of vomiting and some flank pain. She returns, and is sure she has a kidney stone. I do a range of lab and send her for IVP. This is the path of least resistance.

Seventh is a 90-year-old white male with a longstanding esophageal problem for which there is no specific treatment. He's scheduled for feeding tube placement in a couple of days. This will allow him to bypass his esophagus. Now he comes in acutely unable to swallow anything. Even saliva comes back up. He's a keeper. He'll get his feeding tube a day or two early.

Whew...

Our 50-year-old comes back from the ultrasound of his legs, and guess what? They're normal. I call our local oncologist. He tells me that even with a normal ultrasound, he'd put in a filter just because the guy is hypercoagulable (forms blood clots easier than normal). If he doesn't have clot there now, he's proven that he forms clot, and he's sure to have some later. The oncologist tells he that he feels this guy should be shipped to a higher level of care where they can handle these problems.

Then it's time to call back the oncologist and he's NOT happy. I pretty much tell him that all my experts at this end say this guy needs to be at a higher level of care. They tell me he needs to get a Greenfield Filter (a metal filter that goes in the big vein below the heart and catches blood clots), and that they believe it would be inappropriate to try to manage the patient at a facility that cannot offer this procedure. I pretty much hint that if he doesn't accept transfer of his own patient that it borders on patient abandonment. Grudgingly, the guy accepts transfer. Yesss...I arrange a squad to transport, make all the arrangements, and ship him. I've only been working at this about 5 hours!

Our 20-year-old comes back from IVP and it's normal. I can't blame her supposed symptoms on anything I've found so far. At no time has she really even seemed in any real distress. My impression from the beginning was that she, for whatever reason, just wanted to spend the night in the hospital. I send her out. She can follow-up.

Well after that brief interlude, I'm right back at it. The next person is a 60-year-old white male with swelling of his scrotum for a month. He has end stage liver disease with ascites (fluid that collect in the abdomen of folks with bad liver disease). What's happening is that the fluid is tracking down into his scrotum. On this gentleman, his scrotum is about the size of a very large grapefruit. I've seen them the size of footballs, so I'm not too impressed. There's not much to do except support it and try and improve the underlying problem. He's given some reassurance and discharged with follow-up.

A 9-month-old white female with a stuffy nose follows this. It turns out she does have an ear infection. I give her an antibiotic for this and send her out.

The witching hour is approaching, but suddenly I'm without patients. I've got about 50 charts to dictate on, but they can wait. My relief is here, and I notice more worried-well queuing up in the lobby. I am out of here!

I can't go far though. I'm only off for 6 hours, then I'm back for another 18. I call the nursing supervisor, and find an empty hospital bed I can use for the night. It takes me a little bit to wind down, but then I'm out.

12:00 AM

Zzzz...

Shift 4

"Sometimes bad things happen to bad people (not just good ones)!"

Sunday—18 Hours

6:00 AM

Shit, shit, shit…The alarm is going off way too early. I pull my scrubs back on and head downstairs to rejoin the madness. And what do I find? Absolute chaos! Luckily it's chaos winding down rather than chaos revving up. The doc covering my 6-hour reprieve pretty much has everything covered. There are several patients in rooms, but they're either being admitted or discharged. I have all my charts to finish from yesterday. The unit tech has them all stacked in a six-inch tall pile. Oh joy. There's no rest for the wicked.

I'm given a full hour, and work my way through the majority of my stack. Then the worried well start trickling on in. Family went over to pick up grandpa and take him to church when they find he's not doing real well. In this case, they bring their 90-year-old grandfather with right hip pain. It seems he'd fallen 3-4 days ago and is having persistent pain that's making it hard for him to get around, even with his walker. He's in no real distress, so I just send him off for x-ray.

Meanwhile, I see an 80-year-old white female with diarrhea and some low abdominal pain for a week. She's now started having blood in her stools, and complains of hemorrhoids that are "down to her knees." She'd had a colonoscopy (a procedure where the colon is examined with a fiber-optic scope) within the last year, and that was normal, except for a few diverticula.

Diverticula are felt to be one of the evils of the low-fiber western diet. They are little outpouchings in the colon wall that can become inflamed and infected. This leads to (typically) left sided abdominal pain, fever, and occasionally bloody stools. When they are infected, they are treated with antibiotics. Sometimes they require surgery, if they get bad enough or occur frequently enough.

This lady has diffuse lower abdominal tenderness, but nothing real significant. When I go to take a look at her hemorrhoids, I find that she has a rectal prolapse.

Rectal prolapse is a bowel problem that occurs in both the very young and the very old. As folks age, their sigmoid colon and rectum can lose some of its support. Then, when there is straining to have a bowel movement, the distal rectum can essentially turn itself inside out and project through the anus. It looks like a big beefy red mass. Usually you can reduce them by tucking them back in where they belong. In the elderly, they occasionally need surgery if it keeps reccurring.

This patient's prolapse is easily reduced with some mild pressure. Oh the things I do for God and country! I start our standard belly pain work-up. It's likely she's got a flare-up of her diverticulitis as well, but it could easily be something else.

Our 90-year-old guy makes it back and has a pubic rami fracture. The pubic rami is a circle of bones in our pelvis that provides the support when we sit on our bottom. This is considered a stable fracture, and just requires pain control. Then I hear what, on Sunday, are dreaded words from a family, "we just can't manage him at home!" They want him admitted to the hospital.

People just don't understand that we can't admit people to the hospital just because we want to. They must meet specific criteria or their visit will not be paid for. Folks have no concept that just occupying a hospital room can cost $1500 a day, and up! When confronted with this, I usually get such things as, "well, I have insurance," or "well, I have Medicaid." If your insurance or Medicaid is not going to cover it, the question then becomes one of whether the patient or the family is going to. Usually, when they hear the dollar amounts involved, they balk quickly and decide that maybe they can manage grandpa at home after all. Another option can sometimes be a short nursing home stay. This is down around $100-$200 a day, which is a far cry from $1500. However, admission to the nursing home after hours and on weekends is always a challenge, and is frequently impossible. Without supplemental insurance, Medicare or Medicaid rarely covers even nursing homes. I put the wheels in motion to find someplace to put this guy, but its going to take hours.

While all this is going on, I see a 71-year-old white male complaining of weakness. I notice right away that his heart rate is about 30, which is a good reason to be feeling weak. He's had some chest pain last night that resolved with a nitroglycerine tablet, and is having no other complaints at this time. His EKG doesn't really show anything except the slow heart rate. Now the patient is on a couple of medicines that can slow the heart, but they haven't been adjusted recently. We don't have a good cause to think that this guy has over-taken his medicines. This leads me to be suspicious that he has had some type of event that has injured the electrical conduction system of his heart.

The human heart is really multiply redundant when it comes to the mechanisms that keep it beating. There are at least three separate systems that ensure that it keeps going. There's an area high on the heart called the S-A (sinoatrial) node that acts as a pacemaker keeping a resting rate of around 60-100 beats a minute. If this fails, then between the top and bottom of the heart, there's an area called the A-V (atrioventricular) node that kicks in, and usually keeps the heart going at 40-50 beats per minute. If this fails, the ventricles themselves have an intrinsic internal pacing system that keeps them going around 30-40 beats per minute.

This patient was running at a rate that suggests he's lost both his S-A and his A-V nodes. This can happen if folks have a heart attack involving these areas. Now this guy's EKG is normal, but his cardiac enzymes are out of sight. It makes you wonder if the little bit of chest pain he had last night wasn't really a little heart attack. I call his doctor early to get him admitted. Sometimes these folks need pacemakers. We keep crude external pacemakers in the department, but for something definitive, this gentleman needs to be somewhere else.

Next is a 6-year-old white female who's having pain with urination. A urinalysis is done and shows she has a mild urinary infection. She's put on an appropriate antibiotic and sent home.

A 14-month-old white female with fever and congestion follows this. She's got a little ear infection in addition to her cold. She's also put on an antibiotic and sent on her way.

I see a little 80-year-old grandma from the nursing home who has a fever and just "isn't feeling well." She's pretty demented, so I do some veterinary medicine and check out all the systems. I don't really find much. She may have the start of bronchitis. She too is put on an antibiotic and sent packing.

Then there's a 32-year-old white female who twisted her ankle on the ice. Her films are fine. She get routine care, is splinted, and sent on her way.

A common issue faced in the ER follows this. It's a 22-year-old white female who is two months pregnant, has had no prenatal care and is cramping and spotting. Sometimes it's a miscarriage. Roughly 10-15% of all first trimester pregnancies end in spontaneous abortion. Sometimes the patient has something simple like a urinary tract infection. Sometimes she is just having some spotting and cramping that means nothing. And sometimes she is having an ectopic pregnancy. These are just a few of the "sometimes." Any more these days, I just take the path of least resistance, do some basic lab, and send them to ultrasound. All these girls want an ultrasound. They think it's the only way to prove their baby is okay. I send her off to get it done. We'll see...

Let's go back to our little 90-year-old with the pelvic fracture. We've finally managed to find him a spot at one of the local nursing homes. They're making special arrangements to process him in on the weekend. Thank God! Not much later and he's gone.

I also see a 70-year-old white female who "hasn't been able to pee" since last night. I have a bladder scan done (a special ultrasound to measure the amount of urine in the bladder), and there's only about a cup (hardly enough to be concerned about). We have her try to urinate, and she gives us a sample. Grossly, it looks like pus, so it's not too difficult to guess what we're going to find. And surprise! She has a bladder infection. She's put on an antibiotic, some symptomatic medicines, and is sent on her way.

There's a 40-year-old white male who's a bipolar and an alcoholic. He's here with nausea, vomiting, and diarrhea for three days. It's noteworthy that he's bypassed two Emergency Rooms between here and his home. This is always rather suspicious. He's likely either got the stomach bug that's been making the rounds, or the brown-bottle flu (alcoholic gastritis). He's a bit shaky and hypertensive to boot, so it's likely that he's in alcohol withdrawal. I tank him up with some IV fluids, thiamin, Compazine (an anti-nausea medicine), and Zantac (a stomach acid medicine). Then I send him on his way. I didn't give him the option to ask me for a narcotic or to refill the Xanax (a tranquilizer) that he's allegedly on.

This is an appropriate point to have a little social discussion. Alcoholics are frequently deficient in thiamin, and so we routinely supplement them with this vitamin in the ER. Failure to do so can trigger an acute psychosis (Wernicke's encephalopathy) if the alcoholic is fed, or gets glucose either orally or in an intravenous solution. Wernicke's is a progressive neurological condition that can be fatal. The condition could be completely avoided if the alcoholic's beverages of choice (usually cheap alcohol fortified wines) were supplemented with thiamin. However, this is not politically expedient, so it doesn't happen. Therefore, folks either die or have permanent disability for essentially political reasons. This tends to be a politically disenfranchised population, so the situation continues year after year. Ah well...

Our 22-year-old with the cramping makes it back. It looks likes she's got a miscarriage well under way. All these girls want to know what they can do to stop it. Well, the answer is nothing! There really isn't anything that can be done until about the 20th week of gestation. Usually with these first trimester miscarriages it's because there's something wrong with the fetus that is incompatible with life. In this case, it looks like it's a blighted ovum. This is where there is enough genetic material to make the amniotic sac and convince the body it's pregnant, but not enough to actually produce a fetus. She's given something for discomfort, counseled, and sent on her way. She can follow-up tomorrow. Most of these completely abort spontaneously. A small number have continued bleeding and need a D&C (a procedure where they scrape the tissue out of the uterus).

Next I see a 2-month-old white male with a low-grade fever, clear nasal drainage, and fussiness. There's really not much on exam that's noteworthy, and the kid's in no real distress. However, I'm always more conservative on the kids that are under two months old.

Kids less than two months of age are a special case, and are felt to have an incomplete immune system. They are a bit more prone to certain types of infection, some of which can be threatening. Because of this, they are managed much more aggressively than older kids.

With this little guy, I come up with a positive RSV (respiratory syncytial virus) screen. The lay press has consistently terrorized folks about this for years. It's true that a small percentage of kids can develop severe breathing problems with RSV, but for the vast majority it's just a "bad cold." When I say the RSV word, the immediate response of these parents is, "then you're going to admit him, right?" Ah, ...no! The kid is fine, he's having no breathing problems, and his oxygen level is 100%. There's no reason to admit him. I put him on a nebulizer just for good measure, and recommend that they be proactive about having the child seen if he gets worse. I wind up having to spend 20-30 minutes explaining what RSV really is, and how it usually isn't as bad as it's made out to be.

My next victim is a 28-year-old white female who fell on her left arm at work. You would swear someone had cut off her arm the way she's acting. There is no obvious injury and her x-rays are normal. I don't know. It's like the lights are on, but nobody's home with this girl. I put her in a wrist/forearm splint for good measure, and give her routine sprain instructions.

12:00 PM

Lunch sucks. It's hardly worth mentioning. Why is cafeteria food so uniformly disgusting?

The town is waking up, so our lobby is filling up fast. It's our lunchtime crowd.

First I see a 7-year-old white male with a fever and sore throat. He's got a positive strep screen and has strep throat. He gets an antibiotic and is sent on his way.

Second I see a 5-year-old white female with a headache, fever, and stomach upset. She's got an ear infection. She's had some vomiting, so I give her a shot of Rocephin (a broad-spectrum antibiotic). A single shot will cure the vast majority of ear infections.

Third is real winner. It's a 30-year-old white male with 3 weeks of low back pain. He's been seeing a chiropractor, and it's only getting worse. The real twist is that he's noted some swelling of his legs, and now he's convinced he could have blood clots in his legs. The probability of this in an otherwise young, healthy, person is almost zero. However, I send him down for an ultrasound to prove this to him.

Fourth is an 80-year-old white male who's feeling light headed. His blood pressure is a bit on the low side, and he's a little bit anemic. He's also on a handful of blood pressure medicines. He doesn't have any blood in his stools, which makes it less likely that he's bleeding into his gut. I give him some IV fluids, and that makes him feel a bit better. I reduce his water pill for a couple of days, and coordinate follow-up with his regular doctor.

Fifth is an 80-year-old grandma who's had some leg swelling for a month, and an intermittent fever for a week. She's sure that the leg swelling means she has a blood clot. Boy, are they putting something in the water to make these people? She gets some basic lab, and is sent down with our other leg swelling guy for an ultrasound of her legs.

Sixth is an 85-year-old white female with right sided belly pain. She's also allegedly had black stools. Her exam does exhibit some diffuse right-sided pain, but her stool is brown and has no blood in it. I start a routine abdominal pain work-up, and have the nurse give her some IV fluids and a mild pain medicine. We'll see.

Well surprise, surprise. Our folks with the leg swelling both have normal ultrasounds. It turns out that the older lady was recently put on an arthritis medicine that is known to cause leg swelling. I have her stop it and put on something else. She may also have a little virus with the fever she's been having. They can both follow-up as needed.

Seventh is a 8-year-old white male with a sore throat, ear pain, and mattery eyes. His strep screen is negative, but he does have an ear infection as well as an infection of both eyes. He's put on an oral antibiotic and some antibiotic eye drops. He'll need to be rechecked in about a week.

Eighth is a 20-year-old white female with a fever, sore throat, and vomiting. You would swear she was on death's doorstep the way she is acting. I start her on some IV fluids and Compazine (an anti-nausea medicine) and send off a strep screen.

In the 85-year-old with the belly pain, I'm just not finding anything going on. She's sufficiently miserable that I order a CT scan of her abdomen and pelvis just for good measure. She has pain and tenderness in the right upper abdomen that could be consistent with gallbladder disease, but she also has pain in the right lower abdomen that could be an appendicitis or diverticulitis. Add to this the fact that she's had prior abdominal surgeries, and bowel obstruction, adhesions, and the like could come into play. We'll see…

Hmmm. Our 2-year-old with the sore throat and vomiting has strep throat. I have the nurse jab her with long acting penicillin. When she can tolerate oral fluids, she can go.

What a winner! Ninth is a 50-year-old white male who was using his leg for a saw horse and took a skill saw across his thigh. This has got to be the third one of these in the last month! Don't they realize that the saw blade projects below the board when they're cutting it? Talk about stupid! Luckily it's pretty shallow. It takes a couple of dozen stitches, and he's sent on his way.

Boy it seems like for every patient I get out of here, there's two to take their place.

Tenth is a 60-year-old white male with a persistent cough and rib soreness for a week. He does have a few wheezes, and is dramatically improved with a breathing treatment. Surprisingly enough, he isn't a smoker. I put him on an antibiotic and an inhaler and send him off.

Eleventh is a 50-year-old white male with left shoulder pain after moving an large appliance at home. There was no trauma. This guy really just wants a get-out-of-work card. Fine! Whatever.

Twelfth is a 18-year-old white male with nausea and vomiting for the last two days. He's also got right lower abdominal pain. It's not real dramatic, but it's there. His lab is all-normal, but the question of appendicitis has been brought up, so I send him off for a CT scan of his pelvis.

In the meantime, our 85-year-old with the belly pain has returned. It seems she has acute gallbladder disease. It's a rather unusual presentation for that, and the lab sure doesn't point us in that direction. I call her regular doctor and get her admitted. She'll likely loose her gallbladder tomorrow.

Thirteenth is a 16-year-old white female with a sore throat and ear pain. Her strep screen is negative, but she does have an ear infection involving both ears. She gets some antibiotics, and is sent along.

Fourteenth is an 80-year-old white female who had an episode where she couldn't talk for about an hour. She has a stroke history. She's already had one neck artery reamed out, and she's on Coumadin and aspirin (both are blood thinners). This means she's already on maximum medical therapy for stroke prevention. In her case, the two key issues are to make sure her blood is thin enough, and to make sure that she hasn't had a bleed into her brain. I get some lab and send her off to get her brain scanned.

Our 18-year-old with the vomiting and belly pain makes it back from CT. It looks like he does have appendicitis. I call his regular doctor. I imagine he'll probably get it out before the night is through.

Appendicitis is an illness that is actually only rarely seen at large referral hospitals. It's usually picked up at the smaller rural hospitals. A classic presentation is that of a progressive abdominal pain that starts around the belly button, and migrates to the lower right side of the abdomen. There is frequently fever, nausea, and anorexia (not wanting to eat). These symptoms usually progress slowly over a period of a day or so.

It used to be that surgeons were felt to be under-diagnosing appendicitis if they didn't take out normal appendixes at least 25% of the time. However, these days CT has gotten so good that it can correctly diagnose appendicitis about 95% of the time.

Fifteenth is a 45-year-old white male with sinus symptoms for a week. His nose is stuffy and he just can't sleep at night. My heart bleeds for you! I give him a cold pack and send him on his way.

Sixteenth is a 16-year-old white female with several hours of pain and burning with urination. Her urinalysis is strongly positive for infection. She gets an antibiotic and something for discomfort. She'll need to follow-up in a few days to make sure it clears up.

Seventeenth is a 24-year-old white female who cut her thumb while doing the dishes. It's over a joint and gapes whenever she flexes the joint, so I put a couple of stitches into it.

Back to our 80-year-old with the spell where she couldn't talk. Her blood is as thin as it should be. Her blood pressure is normal. Her brain scan doesn't show any bleeding. I chat with her regular doctor and the neurologist. There really isn't anything further to offer her today. She's on every protective medicine we can give her already.

She'll need follow-up tomorrow to rescan her neck and to make sure she doesn't need her neck arteries cleaned out again. She also needs a look-see to make sure there's no other source of clot that could lead to stroke. But there's nothing that's going to be done tonight. Hence, there's no real good reason to admit her to the hospital. She can follow-up with her regular doctor tomorrow and he can honcho the work-up.

6:00 PM

Dinner is re-warmed lunch, and is just as bad.

The people just keep on coming...

Eighteenth is a 6-year-old white female with a fever, sore throat, and vomiting. She has strep throat, but doesn't want a shot. I give her some Phenergan (an anti-nausea medicine), and make sure she can keep stuff down. She goes home with an oral antibiotic and some Phenergan suppositories.

Nineteenth is a 40-year-old white female with neck pain for a week. She has a remote history of a cervical fusion (vertebra in the neck are surgically fused), but there's been no recent trauma. I give her some Toradol (an anti-inflammatory) , some Valium (a tranquilizer used as an anti-spasmodic), and send her to get her neck filmed. Of course it's fine, and she's better. She gets my routine back medicines and is sent away.

Twentieth is a 60-year-old white male with multiple episodes of grossly bloody stools throughout the day. He'd just had a colonoscopy (a lighted fiber optic scope is used to visually inspect the entire colon) within the last couple of months that was essentially normal. I put a finger in his butt and did not pull out a plum, but got a fair amount of gross blood. His blood count is low, so he's losing blood from somewhere in there. I contact his regular doctor, and he's admitted directly.

Twenty-first is a 10-year-old white male with two hours of nausea, vomiting, and diarrhea. He's got the bug that's been going around. He refuses a suppository, and wants a shot instead for his vomiting. His stomach calms down until he is able to keep fluids down, and he is sent on his way.

Twenty-second is a 35-year-old white male who was bit by his dog. He has multiple puncture wounds to his hand. His dog is current on his shots.

The biggest concern with a hand bite in this country is bacterial infection, and not rabies. The dog mouth carries an organism known as Pasteurella Multocida that can cause a bad skin infection.

I clean up this guy's hand and put him on Augmentin (an antibiotic with coverage for Pasteurella) for good measure.

Twenty-third is a 16-year-old white male with a cold for three days. This is really foolish. His family are very frequent visitors to our ER. The mom demands a chest x-ray of her son. Of course it's normal. Hell, I've got a cold and am sicker than this kid is. He can use symptomatic medicines, and he will get better.

Twenty-fourth is an 8-year-old white female with a barky cough. She does seem to be having some problems breathing, although her oxygen level is normal. I have respiratory give her a racemic epinephrine nebulizer treatment (a fast acting short duration breathing medicine). I also give her a whopping dose of Decadron (a steroid). She's got laryngotracheobronchitis, or croup.

Croup is a viral infection that is really a lot less prevalent since the advent of the HiB (Haemophilus Influenza B) vaccination. That bug used to give us a lot of epiglottis, a potentially life threatening airway obstruction produced by inflammation and swelling in the upper airway.

I do a chest and soft tissue neck x-rays on this girl for good measure, and they're fine (there's specific radiographic findings we look for that tell us if croup has progressed to the more threatening epiglotitis). We watch her for a couple of hours to make sure she doesn't rebound and have worsening symptoms. Then we let her go home with some Pediapred (a liquid steroid elixir) and routine croup instructions.

The last case of my shift is actually kind of interesting. It's a 35-year-old white female with several hours of left sided chest pain. The pain is sharp, radiates to the back, and is not changed by movement or breathing. It is, however, improved with leaning forward. This patient has a history of pericarditis in the distant past, and says that it feels just like that.

Pericarditis is an inflammation of the sack that surrounds the heart. It's typically caused either by a viral infection or an autoimmune disease. Occasionally, this can lead to the collection of fluid around the heart that can reach a point where it compromises the hearts ability to pump effectively. It usually responds to anti-inflammatories or steroids, but in rare cases needs either needle aspiration or a surgery to allow collected fluid to drain away from the heart. The surgery is known as a pericardial window. When this is done, an opening is made in the pericardium, allowing collected fluid to drain into the abdomen. Pericarditis usually has characteristic clinical, EKG and laboratory findings.

In this patient I'm coming up empty except for the clinical findings. My relief shows up early though, and I'd rather go home and to bed than satisfy my curiosity. I check it out to him, and hit the road. I actually have several days off in a row. Thank God!

12:00 AM

Shift 5

"Vanishing into the void..."

Saturday—18 Hours

6:00 AM

The last shift has seen only one patient since last evening at 11:00 PM. Wouldn't you know it, I'm here less than 60 seconds and someone drives into our squad bay and demands immediate attention for their family member. In addition, someone else is checking into through the lobby, and a nursing home calls to tell us they're sending someone along as well.

And here we go...

My first case of the day is a 65-year-old white male with a known lung cancer. He's having cancer pain that is not adequately controlled with his current medicines. This person looks like he just came over from a concentration camp. He's had problems with a recurrent pleural effusion (fluid from the tumor collecting under, and collapsing the lung), and was recently sclerosed (a irritating compound, like talc or tetracycline, is infused into the area where fluid keeps reaccumulating in an attempt to adhere the lung to the chest wall). All these things are red flags to me. It tells me that this cancer is terminal (not exactly rocket science). It also brings up an interesting point about cancer patients and pain control.

This is perhaps as good a point as to talk about pain management, especially pain management in the cancer patient. Many doctors are reluctant to adequately control their cancer patient's pain. These folks can frequently take huge doses of narcotics to even begin to get comfortable. There is reluctance, on the part of the doctors, to give the doses required. They're worried about addiction, the DEA (Drug Enforcement Agency) auditing their prescribing practices, whatever. This means that a lot of these folks show up in the ER very uncomfortable and very unhappy with their regular doctor.

In this case, I use the pain medicine the patient is already taking as a starting point to begin to get him comfortable. I give him a substantial dose of Morphine (a strong narcotic) and wait to see how it's going to work...

Meanwhile, I check out a 57-year-old white female with recurrent vague left-sided chest pain for a week. Her regular doctor thinks it's reflux (stomach acid bubbling up into her esophagus), but it hasn't been responding her reflux medicines.

There is also a 16-year-old white male with 4 days of fever, body aches, cough, and ear pain. Of course it's an emergency this morning. He couldn't be bothered to see his regular doctor any time in the last four days. I do an influenza screen that is negative. He does have an ear infection. Otherwise, he's got the viral creeping crud. I put him on an antibiotic, some symptomatic medicines, and send him on his way.

Our 65-year-old cancer patient we've gotten comfortable. He has reaccumulated some fluid under his lung, but it's not making him short of breath. His oxygen level is fine. I rearrange his pain medicines. If he gets more short of breath, we can drain his chest, but for now we can just keep an eye on it. He can follow-up first of the week.

I've also got a 70-year-old white female who had fallen at the nursing home and complains of right ankle pain. On x-ray she has a non-displaced distal fibula fracture (the bone on the outside of the ankle). She's put in a walking boot (an orthopedic support boot used in this type of fracture), and given a walker. She can follow-up first of the week.

Our 57-year-old with the vague chest pain has completely normal lab and EKG. She's had no symptoms throughout her stay, and is considered low risk. I discuss it with her regular doctor, and she can follow-up first of the week.

I see a 24-year-old white female with a rash where she'd had some surgical tape. It's an emergency rash! This is an obvious contact dermatitis (like you get with poison oak or poison ivy) in an area about a quarter inch square. I give her a little stronger topical steroid than is available over the counter, and send her on her way.

I also see a 90-year-old white male who had struck his right elbow on the toilet a few days ago. He's complaining of elbow pain and swelling. The x-ray shows no obvious fracture, but he's got some soft findings of a radial head fracture (the bone in the elbow that aids in our ability to rotate our wrist). This warrants a sling, an anti-inflammatory, a pain pill, and follow-up. Even with a through and through fracture, it's one that doesn't normally require a cast.

Boy we are just stomping out disease and pestilence!

Next is a 90-year-old white female with left ear pain off and on for the last several days. She comes in today because the weather is projected to be getting worse later today. There's a significant amount of snow in the forecast. She's decided to come in now, as she doesn't want to run the risk of having to come in later when the weather is worse. She's got a bit of infection in the ear canal, and is put on some antibiotic drops to fix this.

Then we have a common problem for the weekend. It's a 55-year-old white female with a recent colon cancer, who's getting adjuvant chemotherapy. She's been having nausea, vomiting, and diarrhea for at least the last week. She's relatively dehydrated, and that's the biggest risk. We do some basic lab, start some IV fluids, and give her some Zofran (a anti-nausea medicine that works best for chemotherapy associated vomiting). Usually it's just a matter of tanking these folks up. However, it's likely to be an ongoing problem as long as she's on chemo. The alternative to chemo is death, so there aren't very many good options.

This is followed by a work-related injury that's pretty common. It's a 50-year-old white female, factory worker, with pain and numbness in her fingers and radiating up her arm. This has been coming on for several weeks.

This is pretty classic for carpal tunnel disease. Carpal tunnel is a disorder that mostly affects folks who use their hands a lot. It's in the category of repetitive motion injury. You wind up with inflammation of the big nerve in the wrist, the median nerve. This produces numbness and pain in the thumb and adjacent two fingers as well as half of the ring finger. The other half of the ring ringer and the pinkie get sensation from a different nerve entirely, the ulnar nerve. Carpal tunnel is usually confined to palm surfaces, as the back of the hand gets sensation from yet another nerve, the radial nerve.

The median nerve is the only nerve in the wrist at significant risk as it passes through a fairly tightly enclosed space there in the wrist.

This disorder frequently responds to simple things, like anti-inflammatory medicines. It's position and use related, so a second line of attack can be a wrist splint worn either overnight or while working. If these maneuvers don't work, there is a surgery that can be done, a carpal tunnel release, where a ligament is transected in the wrist, giving more space for the nerve.

It seems to be a morning for hand problems. Next is a 38-year-old white male who jammed his finger at work. You would swear he had cut it off given the way he's acting. His x-ray is normal. He's sent off with symptomatic medicines

Argggg…It's my favorite. NOT! Next is a 30-year-old white female who tells me she wants to kill herself. She has a long history of suicidal thoughts, and has decided she want to go back to the local psychiatric hospital. What an ordeal this is! At least she's not kicking and screaming, but wants to go. I have her blood alcohol drawn, and get a pregnancy test. These are pretty much the minimum that the psych boys want before they will accept a patient. I also have the local police called so we can get an emergency hold on this girl. This is the only way she can be held against her will for psychiatric evaluation. With all of this stuff done, we start making the calls to get her a psychiatric evaluation...

Psychiatric care out of the Emergency Room can be almost impossible. The real problem is usually one of money. Most of the folks with severe psychiatric problems are uninsured and uninsurable. Of course no psychiatrist wants to take patients who have no means of paying their bills.

Here locally, if a patient comes in making suicidal statements or gestures, we can at least get the local police to put a hold on them. Then, in this county at least, the county picks up the tab to get them an inpatient evaluation.

Unfortunately, these patients are frequently lost to follow-up when they get out of the psychiatric hospital, at least until they come and see us the next time.

12:00 PM

And wouldn't you know it, now is when we get our next squad. It's an 88-year-old white female who was found unresponsive at the local nursing home. She's in a pretty deep coma, and will just twitch slightly to painful stimulus. She's at least protecting her airway. Also, and most importantly, she comes with the magic DNR (Do Not Resuscitate) forms.

Advance directives are so frequently overlooked by people. If you're elderly and have a range of medical conditions, most of which cannot be fixed, you and your family need to be realistic about what and how much medical intervention should be done if you wind up in a medical crisis. The reality is that often as much as 90% of the lifetime medical resources expended on a patient occurs in the last couple of weeks of their life. This sort of investment may be justified if there is some reasonable hope of turning the situation around, but so frequently there is nothing definitive that can be done. We end up torturing these folk, giving them painful and protracted deaths. The reality is that everyone is going to die sometime. I believe that if folks have got to die, they are at least entitled to a peaceful death.

So much for my rant! With this lady, rather than asking "what's going on?" a better question is "what's not going in?" As the objective information starts coming in, it looks like she's had a stroke, a heart attack, is in heart failure, has dangerously low sodium levels, etc, etc. She's working pretty hard to die. I do some simple, and relatively inexpensive interventions, with oxygen, Lasix (a water medicine), Lovenox (a blood thinner), and nitroglycerine paste. I also call her regular doctor early so he can take over this mess. In the end, I'll be surprised if she survives the day, let alone to discharge from the hospital.

And now we go to more mundane stuff. I see a 19-year-old white female complaining of sore throat and headache. This is yet another example of high drama. Her exam is normal. Her strep test is negative. Despite this, she still wants and antibiotic. I give her a course of Amoxicillin and send her on her way.

A 90-year-old white female follows this. She comes in by squad from the nursing home. She has had a cough for the last several days, and has an intermittent sharp left sided chest pain when she coughs. The nursing home staff somehow seems convinced that these cold symptoms represent a cardiac event. More to appease the nursing home, I do an EKG. Of course, it's completely normal. Given the patient's age, I do a chest x-ray. It too is normal. All the while, this little lady is wondering why she's even here. In the end, I cover her with an antibiotic, and give her a cough medicine. She then goes back to the nursing home (what she wanted in the first place).

We are back then to one of our frequent fliers. It's a 22-year-old white female who we see frequently with "migraine headache." Of course today is no different than her past visits. She tells me this is MUCH worse than her usual headache. She states that "this is the worst one ever," though this is what she tells me pretty much every time. I always ask myself when dealing with these folks, why is this headache always the worst one? I've never had a very good answer. A real problem is that these folks cry wolf so frequently that, if they were indeed having their fatal subarachnoid bleed, no one would believe them. At least she doesn't ask me for a narcotic. She seems to accept what I give her. She's given one of my usual concoctions consisting of Nubain, Phenergan, and DHE-45. She may not go way happy, but she goes away.

Again high drama is the order of the day when the next patient arrives. It's a 38-year-old white female who arrives by squad after three minutes of sharp left-sided chest pain. This pain is worse with movement and a deep breath. She is convinced that she is having a heart attack. She has no other associated symptoms. She has no cardiac risk factors. The initial impression is that she is having a serious panic attack. Of course her EKG is completely normal as is every other tests that's done. She's completely cured with a dose of Toradol (an anti-inflammatory) and Xanax (a tranquilizer). Perhaps the most time con-suming aspect of the whole ordeal is convincing her that she's going to be all right. It doesn't help that she has both a significant psychiatric history as well as a drug abuse history. In the end, I prevail and get her out the door.

Psychiatric cases appear to be the order of the day, and the next patient is no exception to this rule. It's a 19-year-old white male visit-ing us for the second time in less than 24 hours with flu symptoms. His level of drama was so extreme on his previous visit that the physician on duty at that time did the $2,000 work-up. Of course everything was normal on that exam. He was felt to have a viral syndrome, and was advised to use over the counter medicines to treat this symptomati-cally. The patient is here today because he is just "no better." He also states that he is both weak and short of breath. Now, the patient does have asthma, is a smoker, and has "lost" his inhaler.

This is a point where we're on the horns of a dilemma. The unwrit-ten law in these cases where folks have had a significant work up and subsequently returned is that you always do more on the second visit. This is more medicolegal than strictly medical. In this patient's case, I order everything but the kitchen sink, knowing it's all going to be pretty much normal. In addition, perhaps the one definitive thing I do is to give the patient a breathing treatment. As for the rest of the studies, we'll see...

Meanwhile, I see a 69-year-old white male who had a recent rectal surgery and for the last 12 hours has been unable to pee. As you might imagine, he looks pretty uncomfortable. This gentleman does have a history of prostate gland problems, and has had a transurethral prostate resection (the rotor rooter job you hear about) in the past. He also relates that he's had some burning with urination for the last several days. This suggests some combination of either infection or prostate problem. The quickest way to tell the story is to just put at catheter into his bladder. This is done and quickly drains over a quart of urine. A sample of his urine is sent to a laboratory, but it's normal. Sometimes the stress of a surgery combined with pain medicine can be enough to make a borderline prostate problem more apparent. I'll leave the catheter in place for the weekend, and he can follow-up with his urologist on Monday.

This is followed directly by a 21-year-old white male with hives. He's had no specific new exposures, and he's tried nothing for the symptoms. As I commented elsewhere, this tends to be an allergic reaction to something either ingested or inhaled. In this patient's case, his symptoms are very minimal. They consist of a few patches of itchy red rash. If he had the forethought to call his regular physician, he would have either been advised to take some Benadryl or he might have had a script called in. In his case, I give him a shot of Decadron (a steroid) and Visteril (an antihistamine). I also give him a prescription for Atarax (an oral equivalent of Visteril). One of the rules of the emergency room is that, where possible, the patient needs to go home with the cure.

Back to our 19-year-old with the flu symptoms. As expected, everything comes back normal. He does indeed have a viral syndrome. It would've been nice if I could have found that he had influenza. I then would have been able to send him home with one of the antiviral medications that treat this virus. Unfortunately, I really don't find anything. Though the patient doesn't think so, he's going to live. I give him a new Combivent inhaler, and reemphasize that he has a benign self-limited illness that requires only symptomatic treatment. I volunteer a doctor's note to get him out of work for the next couple of days. When all is said and done, this is likely his original agenda.

Next is a 45-year-old white female with red itchy burning mattery eyes for last three to four days. She's a patient of doctor NONE, who figured that if she waited long enough it would go way. She didn't want to see a physician because she has no insurance, and didn't want to incur the expense. This has turned a $30 office visit into a $300 emergency room visit. She's got a world-class case of conjunctivitis (pinkeye). In addition, she tells me she has no money to buy medicine. She does, however, have enough money to buy cigarettes. In a momentary act of kindness, I round up a bottle of antibiotic eyedrops from our stock and send her on her way.

Shortly thereafter, I see a 21-year-old white male with a laceration on his right hand. Apparently, he was trying to capture a wasp with a glass jar. He slammed the jar down, it shattered, and the rest is history. You would think he would've come up with a better story. It's a fairly superficial laceration, but it does require suturing. Ten stitches later and he's out the door.

Then, thankfully, we have something real. It's a 50-year-old white female who has a history of breast cancer. She's had a mastectomy, but because of advanced disease is requiring adjuvant chemotherapy and radiation therapy. With each bout of chemotherapy she has problems with nausea and vomiting. She's been trying to manage this at home with pills and suppositories, but has been unable to keep it under control. This is a very common problem where we can intervene effectively, usually intravenous fluids and antiemetics (typically Zofran, an antiemetic that works well with chemotherapy). I start the fluids, push the drugs, and wait to see how she does.

Surprise, two real cases in a row! This time it's a 45-year-old white female with right upper abdominal pain. She's had this off and on for the last one to two weeks, but today it's been much worse. In reality, this is a pretty cut and dried case. This patient qualifies as a 40-year-old fat, fertile, female, and these are the classic risk factors for gallbladder disease. She does seem pretty uncomfortable. I have my nurse start an IV, and give her some Demerol (a narcotic). This should keep her comfortable while we do the work-up. I order my standard abdominal pain lab, and wait for the results.

In the meantime, it's back to foolishness. This is in the form of an 8-year-old white female who has fallen at home and bumped her head. There was no loss of consciousness, she's been appropriate since, and she has no specific complaints. She has a very small bruise on her forehead. Her mother raced her out to the emergency room because of the bruise. She has the small bruise, and that's it. It really has me scratching my head. Sometimes I just don't understand people. I spend 10 to 15 minute providing reassurance, and send them on their way with head injury instructions.

The next case, though it starts out rather poorly, actually evolves into something real. It's a 48-year-old white female with severe asthma and uncontrolled diabetes. She is also one of our frequent fliers, and it doesn't help that she's a chronic alcoholic. Today she comes in complaining that she feels short of breath and is shaky. This is a case where my prior comment about crying wolf has some substance. This patient has been in the Emergency Department dozens of times with similar complaints, but rarely is it anything serious. My initial feeling is that this is a similar visit, but I try to be complete in my evaluation of each patient regardless of what I might think of them personally. Perhaps cruelly, as a form of punishment, I order a set of arterial blood gases. This is a moderately painful procedure were a needle is put into the artery in the wrist and blood is withdrawn; it is the Gold Standard for measuring blood oxygen. Respiratory therapy tries several times, but are unable to obtain a sample. They ask if I will try. My attempt constitutes the sixth or seventh try, but I managed to get it immediately. Meanwhile, the patient is given a breathing treatment. Surprisingly, when the blood gases returned, they are awful. The patient needs to be on supplemental oxygen. By itself, this constitutes admission criteria for hospitalization. The chest x-ray and the other laboratory are essentially normal.

This likely constitutes severe exacerbation of the patient's asthma. It turns out she has been drinking heavily for at least a day, and the shakiness is likely early alcohol withdrawal. I call the doctor on call for her regular physician, and arrange for her to be admitted.

Getting back to our 50-year-old cancer patient, she's feeling significantly better and is ready to leave. As for our 45-year-old with the abdominal pain, her liver enzymes are elevated consistent with acute gallbladder disease. She is sent for ultrasound, and it's completely consistent with this. Actually, before I have all the results back, I am so confident with my diagnosis that I contact her regular physician and arrange for her admission.

On the scanner it sounds like there's a squad out. There seems to be car wreck after car wreck out on the ice. We have our first group inbound from the latest conflagration.

I still have a few minutes, so I see a 24-year-old white female who presents with neck pain. This patient has a significant history of neck injury and subsequent repair. She has had several herniated disks that required surgical repair. The patient is having increasing problems with neck pain. To do further surgery will render her incapable of turning her head from side to side. To avoid this, her doctors have been trying epidurals (this is where steroid and pain medicine is injected around the nerve roots in the neck in an attempt to control pain). The patient had this procedure done just a few days ago, and is having a significantly increased pain. Her doctors are apparently giving her injectable Demerol (a big gun narcotic) for her to use at home. She tells me that she ran out of her Demerol, and is unable to make arrangements for refills on the weekend. Of course this sounds a very suspicious. This is a typical ploy of our drug seeking clientele in their attempt to convince us to give them the narcotic of their choice. This is a judgment call. I'm able to verify the bulk of her story, and note that she isn't a frequent visitor to our Emergency Department. She has physical exam findings consistent with her specified surgery and that is suggestive of significant neck spasm. I tell her that I am uncomfortable giving her more injectable Demerol, but that I am willing to give her an oral equivalent in quantities sufficient to get her through the weekend. This is acceptable to her and in fact is what she prefers. I calculate an equivalent amount of oral Demerol to what she had been injecting and give her a prescription for 10 pills.

Moments later, the fun begins. The squads begin arriving. First is a 55-year-old morbidly obese white male, a patient of doctor NONE, with neck and back pain. He was a restrained passenger in the front seat when his car was struck and from behind at a stoplight. There is very little damage to the car. The interior of the car is intact. The patient comes in on a backboard with a cervical collar in place. This is likely just a neck sprain, but I am obligated to prove that there is no significant in jury. Therefore I order x-rays of the neck and upper back.

6:00 PM

Meanwhile I see another of the communities finest. It's a 44-year-old white male who months ago had punched his fist through a window and embedded glass in his hand. He's convinced that there's a piece of glass left in his hand, and demands that we remove it. Of course, this is another patient who works at UNEM, is insured by SELF, and a patient of doctor NONE. I'm sure this patient doesn't realize that by coming to the Emergency Department to have this looked at he's going to receive a bill for $500 to $700, or more. This might compare to a similar office visit where the issue could be addressed at a cost of perhaps 20 percent of that. I'm not convinced that there is glass where the patient thinks there is. Indeed, when I explore his hand, all I find is some scar tissue. He seems happy that I looked, but I'm sure this will change when he gets the bill.

From there I see a 9-month-old Hispanic female who's been pulling at her ear. She's had a low-grade fever and increasing fussiness for last couple of days. Her left eardrum is infected. I put her on Amoxicillin and send her on her way.

This is followed immediately by a 6-year-old white female who's been having pain with urination through the day. Her nurse has obtained a urinalysis prior to my exam, and it's completely normal.

Therefore, I round up the nurse for the exam. In the absence of a urinary tract infection, I need to look for other causes of this patient's
symptoms. Young girls are especially uncomfortable with strange men
looking at their privates. Having a nurse present makes it easier and
minimizes legal risk. In this case, I find a very irritated looking yeast
infection. I start the patient on some Lotrisone, and at the mother's
insistence provide some Tylenol with codeine elixir (a mild narcotic).

By this time our 55-year-old motor vehicle accident victim is back
from Radiology. Of course everything is normal. I put him on some
symptomatic medicines and send him on his way.

I then see another of doctor NONE's patients. It's a 40-year-old
white male with recurrent back pain and sinus symptoms for the last
month. He's convinced he has a urinary tract infection and a sinus
infection. This obligates us to do a urinalysis, which is normal. The
patient has a specific agenda, and expects to walk out the door with a
script for erythromycin. In keeping with our McMedicine policy, I give
him what he wants.

Another squad arrives with a 2-year-old white female who bumped
her forehead on some furniture at home. In addition, she sustained a
very minimal scratch to her eyelid. Her parents completely decompen-
sated and called the squad. The injuries are so minimal, that I examine
the child, and discharge her before the paramedics are out the door.

Hmmm, yet another squad on the scanner is inbound.

First though, there's an 18-year-old white female who had some
dental work yesterday. She was started on Darvocet for pain, and is
now puking her guts out. Given the total picture, this is likely a
Darvocet side effect. I talk her into some intravenous fluids and vomiting medicine. This is likely to get her feeling better the quickest.

This is rich! The family of our 2-year-old was following behind the
squad when they were involved in a near head-on collision. It turns
out they're both inbound themselves by squad.

First to arrive is the mother. She's a 20-year-old white female and
was the restrained passenger. Despite being restrained, she managed to
star the windshield. Surprisingly, she was not knocked unconscious.

She is, of course, on a backboard with a cervical collar in place. Except for a sore forehead and some facial abrasions, she has no complaints. Given that she did star the windshield, I am obligated to do a CT scan of her head and x-rays of her neck. In short order, she vanishes into the Radiology Department.

This allows me time to see a 19-year-old white female with several days of intermittent dizziness. In addition, she's had some cold symptoms. Her exam is completely unremarkable. In a 19-year-old, the most common cause of intermittent dizziness is a viral labyrinthitis. This is a viral infection of the labyrinthian system (the system that allow us to tell up from down) in the inner ear. It is usually self-limited, but there are some symptomatic medications that can be used that sometimes help. I give her one of these, some Antivert, to try. I then send her on her way.

I then have yet another dire emergency, a 38-year-old white female with three to four weeks of nonproductive cough. It is yet another head scratcher as to why this is an emergency today. Her symptoms had begun as a normal cold, but the cough has persisted. She obviously has a post-viral syndrome. This can follow any respiratory illness. Given her concern, I do a chest x-ray, and as expected, it's normal. There is nothing to do for this except treat it symptomatically. It will get better. I put her on some stronger placebo medicines and send her on her way.

By this time, the 24-year-old white male driver of our MVA arrives by squad. He has some minimal neck pain, but otherwise no injuries. Of course he too is on a backboard with a cervical collar in place, and so he quickly joins his wife in Radiology.

Yet another doctor NONE patient awaits. It's a 15-month-old white male who last evening had a fever. The family is sure that the patient has pneumonia, because he's had pneumonia in the past when he had a fever. The child is without symptoms at time of exam, and has a completely normal exam. Despite this, the family is insistent on lab and chest x-ray. The better part of valor is to just do what they want. It saddens me that I am so frequently pressed by family to torture children with unnecessary lab tests, and to expose them to unnecessary radiation. I do what is demanded, and as expected, it's all-normal. Even with this, the family is still skeptical. I try to provide reassurance, but who knows how well it sinks in.

By this time, our car wreck family is back from Radiology. All the films are fine. It requires some time to pick out the glass and clean up the abrasions, but they are finally ready to leave with their child. It is interesting to note that their gross overreaction to a mild injury to their child almost resulted in that child being without parents. Sometimes I just have to shake my head.

My next case is a 6-year-old white male with an emergency sore throat and cough. He's in absolutely no distress. He does have a fever, and also complains of some diffuse body aches. Because of this, I order both a strep and influenza screen. Surprisingly enough, they're both positive. I put the child on some Amoxicillin (an antibiotic) for the strep throat, and some Amantadine (an antiviral) for the influenza. I also provide a stronger cough medicine.

Sore throats are all the rage this evening. Next is a 21-year-old white male with a sore throat for a week. The nurse did a strep screen that is negative. Despite this, the patient still wants an antibiotic. I give him what he wants with the caveat that it may not provide improvement. With this viral pharyngitis, it will get better in a half-dozen days with the antibiotic, or six days without.

At last, something real! It's a 32-year-old white female with increasing leg pain and swelling for the last day. There has been no trauma. The real concern is that she may have a spontaneous blood clot in her leg. Her only real risk factor is that she's on birth control pills. This has a very small associated increased risk of blood clots, especially in smokers. I send her off to Radiology to get an ultrasound of the leg.

Blood clots in the leg, by themselves, are not the primary concern. However, the big vessels there drain back to the right heart and then to the lungs. If a clot breaks off and lodges in the lungs it can produce a range of problems up to and including sudden death. I've had several patients in the Emergency Room who have had this happen. They've gone on to die right in front of me despite my best efforts. That's why this is not to be taken lightly.

Meanwhile, we return to the benign. I see a 3-year-old white male with a sore throat for a day. His strep test is negative and his exam is normal. I manage to convince the parents that he does not need an antibiotic, and that this can be treated symptomatically.

A 13-year-old white female with two days of cough and congestion follows this. She is as dramatic as a 13-year-old can be. Her exam is normal, and an influenza screen is negative. I give her some stronger symptomatic medicines and send her away.

I also see a 3-year-old white male with a low-grade fever for the day. As with the previous child, the exam is normal. The parents have not bothered to give the child Tylenol or Motrin. He has a viral syndrome that warrants symptomatic treatment.

By this time our 32-year-old with a swollen leg is back from her ultrasound. All the major veins in her leg are full of blood clot. The patient is going to need to be on a blood thinner for the next six months at the very least. I contact her regular physician and pass off care.

I then see another actual emergency. It's a 90-year-old white female from one of the local nursing homes with progressive shortness of breath. She looks like she's on death's doorstep. Luckily she comes of that important piece of paper, the DNR (Do Not Resuscitate). I get her on some oxygen, and get the evaluation started. On exam, she appears to be in heart failure, so I get some Morphine and Lasix on board as well. Though it may seem counterintuitive to give a pain medicine to a person in heart failure, it actually has a good rationale. Morphine acts to relax blood vessels allowing them to hold a lot more volume. This has the effect of immediately reducing the load on the heart, and improving the symptoms of patients in heart failure with pulmonary edema (fluid in the lungs). The Lasix will allow excess salt, and thereby fluid, to be excreted by the kidneys providing the same overall result. However, this effect takes quite a bit longer. With these simple measures the patient is quickly feeling better. As the objective information comes available, it supports the initial diagnosis. Her regular physician is contacted and she is whisked up to the hospital floor.

More patients are signing in, but the witching hour approaches. Thankfully, my relief is early and seems eager to get started. I leave the watch to him, and head upstairs to the hospital room that I've staked out for myself. I'm due back in roughly six hours for another 18 hours stretch, so it's time for some power sleeping.

12:00 PM

Zzzz...

Shift 6

"Boredom is a good thing! "

Sunday—18 Hours

6:00 AM

Talk about strange dreams…There must be something about sleeping in a hospital bed that gives you weird dreams. Ah well…

The overnight guy had one patient left that he finished up, otherwise the slate is clear. It sounds like it was pretty busy over night despite the ice storm.

A six-inch tall stack of charts sits on my table to be dictated. How depressing! I know I can't leave tonight until everything is done, so this gives me some grudging motivation to get started…

Three hours later, and I complete the last chart. I am amazed that I've managed this with few disruptions. I'm sure that at any moment the floodgates are going to open.

In this time frame I only see one person, an 80-year-old white male who has a suprapubic catheter (a catheter through the lower abdominal wall into the bladder). He had prostate cancer in the past, and received radiation therapy for this. Since then, he has been unable to urinate normally. His catheter is plugged, and he needs it replaced.

This is a simple procedure, one that the patient could probably do himself, and it's accomplished in about 3 minutes. You use a syringe to deflate a balloon on the end of the catheter, pull the old one out, slip a new one in, and re-inflate the balloon. It's an interesting point that this trivial task will actually generate about 30-45 minutes worth of documentation. An interesting and efficient system that we've got, don't you think?

No sooner is my dictation complete than the fun begins. I see a 20-year-old white female who's completely crazy. She's pregnant with her third child and has about a million complaints. She complains of bleeding, cramping, back pain, being emotional, and vomiting. She'd banged her arm a couple of days ago and also complains of elbow pain. She is just wild, fairly well bouncing from wall to wall. It makes you wonder if she isn't either in the manic phase of bipolar disorder or on methamphetamine. We'll check all this stuff out and see what we find. Of course this patient works at UNEM, sees doctor NONE, and her insurance carrier is SELF. So, I treat her like I'd threat any other patient. We're likely to eat $1000-$1500 in charges before we're done. C'est La Vie.

I also see a 5-year-old hispanic female who's had a sore throat and has felt warm for the last day. Her exam is normal. Her strep and influenza screens are negative. She just needs symptomatic meds. Of course all this must be relayed through an interpreter.

Then we get a real case. It's a 79-year-old white male with twenty minutes of crushing chest pain that radiates into his arms. This started while he was driving. He relates he's been having more frequent chest pain for the last several weeks and has not discussed this with his regular doctor. An EKG is done that shows prominent segment changes consistent with ischemia. These are new changes since his most recent EKG last month. At a minimum, this is unstable angina, and could even be a little heart attack. I start our regular chest pain protocol, and he is rapidly pain free on the standard medicines. This is a good thing. His regular doctor is contacted within minutes of him hitting the door, and he shows up in time to send the guy up to the Intensive Care Unit.

In the middle of this, there is a 34-year-old white male with a red itchy rash just minutes after taking some generic ibuprofen. It doesn't take a rocket scientist to make the association between the two. This is an allergic reaction to something in the pill. He's given some Decadron (a steroid) and some Visteril (an antihistamine), and sent out with some Atarax (an oral antihistamine). He should probably avoid the ibuprofen in the future.

12:00 PM

Hmmm…It seems to be a bit "slow" today. Heaven help me I just used the "S" word. What this usually means is that I'm going to pay later.

All right, I see a 30-year-old white female who's sure she's dying. She's had a cough, congestion, body aches, hoarseness, fatigue, and sore throat for the last two weeks. She bypassed the ER in her own town, and traveled the better part of an hour just to visit us. Don't I feel special? I guess we must be the Mecca. Who knows? After two weeks, why this is an emergency today, I can't really say. I'll do a few tests just out of academic interest, but somehow I don't feel I'm going to come up with anything.

…And the answer is…nada. I can't find zilch on this girl. She's got the bad bug. So she needs to do like everyone else and get plenty of rest, fluids, and the like.

Then we have a run of foolish stuff. There's a 19-year-old white female with a sore throat and a headache. Her strep screen is negative. She's got a virus that she needs to treat symptomatically.

There's also a 92-year-old white female with a cough for a couple of days. I do a chest x-ray just because of her age, but she'll probably out-live me. I put her on an antibiotic for good measure.

There's a 25-year-old white male with a "migraine headache." He comes in by squad because he couldn't get a ride. I give him my usually headache concoction and send him on his way. What a waste of resources!

Oh, not to forget our suicidal person. After two hours of phone calls, we finally get approval to ship her to the funny farm. She's out of here, with a police escort, of course.

Then we get a 40-year-old white female with 5 minutes of sharp left-sided chest pain. This is worse with movement and deep breathing. She's sure she's having a heart attack. Of course everything is normal. She has a bit of pleurisy that is cured with Toradol (an anti-inflammatory). She's also worked herself into a panic attack and is hyperventilating to beat the band. It takes forever to get her calmed down and out the door.

Another winner is a 23-year-old white male with flu symptoms. He has a cough, sore throat, body aches, and "just feels weak." He was in just last night with the same symptoms. He had a $1000 work-up that found nothing. Well today he gets a $1500 work-up, and I know from the start that we'll find nothing. This is a big macho dude. Why are these guys such wimps?

I'm pretty much obligated on a second visit, unless it's completely frivolous, to do more than on the first visit. Again, it's more of a legal issue than a medical issue. If I miss something, it's pretty hard to convince the court I took the patient seriously if I just pat them on the back and say, "Get out of here, you're fine!"

Well, of course, everything is completely normal. He has a virus, just like the doctor told him yesterday. I act compassionate for 30 minutes and try to convince him he's going to live. Ultimately, he hits the road. At last!

The excitement never stops! I see a 26-year-old white male who cut his thumb with a knife at home. This is something a Band-Aid would take care of, and any sensible person would realize that. This gentleman is convinced that he needs stitches, and so I toss in three just to make him happy.

Next is 19-year-old patient of Doctor NONE. He's had a cough for three weeks, and of course, he refuses to admit that his two pack a day smoking habit could be at all to blame. In addition, he's had some vomiting through the morning, and it seems there was trace blood in what he vomited. He acts like he really doesn't want to be here (So why did he come? Who knows?), and he definitely has a very big chip on his shoulder. He's only marginally cooperative with anything we do, and everything we do is normal. He's surely got an acute on chronic bronchitis that is made worse by his smoking. He's also got the stomach bug that's been making the rounds, and has likely irritated his esophagus with his vomiting. I put him on an antibiotic for his (viral) bronchitis, and some Zantac (an acid blocker) plus a nausea pill for his stomach problem.

I really have a hard time understanding cigarette addiction. That something can have you by the balls so completely, that you can't go for more than some a few hours without a fix, is just a mystery to me. I'm also baffled how anyone could think that sucking smoke into his or her lungs is a desirable thing. It's yet another of life's little mysteries that has me completely baffled.

My next patient is a 3-year-old white male who allegedly has had a barky cough for the last several hours. I have a cold, and I'm sicker than this kid. The parents want aggressive treatment, so I put him on a taper of steroids.

Then I see a 12-year-old white male who was trying out some exercise equipment in the local sport Shop, lost his balance, and rapped his chin. He managed a nice laceration for his troubles. Four sutures and he's on his way.

This is followed directly by a 25-year-old white male, a frequent ER visitor, with an alleged "migraine headache." I give him my usual, and kick him out the door.

My next patient is a nut with a capital "N." She is another patient from Doctor NONE, who works at UNEM, and is insured by SELF. This is a 28-year-old white female who states that she's pregnant, and has been having vaginal spotting and lower abdominal cramping for two weeks. She was seen in another emergency room last night, and didn't like what they had to say. She is sexually active, and has not kept her Depo-Provera (a three month birth control medicine) shot up to date. She was last due for this about a month ago. She's been on no other form of birth control. Three weeks ago she had a positive pregnancy test at home. She's here today because she wants an ultrasound. I start from ground zero in this case, and treat it like I would approach any other similar first-trimester patient who's bleeding.

First trimester of bleeding has a very specific work-up. Perhaps as many as 10% or 15% of all first trimester pregnancies end in spontaneous abortion. This is not because the patient's done anything wrong, this is just the basic statistics. Usually it means that there was something fundamentally flawed in the fetus. In these cases, there are a range of possibilities that need to be considered. This runs the gamut from urinary tract infections, miscarriage, ectopic pregnancy, pelvic inflammatory disease, and appendicitis. Therefore, we do a complete exam including a pelvic exam, a range of laboratory tests, and frequently a pelvic ultrasound.

In this patient, her exam is completely unremarkable. I order the routine lab and await the outcome.

In the meantime, I see a 29-year-old white male who's twisted his knee while playing basketball. He's weight bearing without difficulty, and has minimal pain. He is here at the insistence of his friends. I get a film that, of course, is normal. This complements a normal exam. Following the advice of his friends is likely going to cost him about $400. Some friends, huh? In the end, he is discharged with routine sprain instructions.

This is followed by a 39-year-old white female, yet another of our frequent fliers, with yet another "migraine headache." She gets my standard concoction and is kicked out the door.

At long last, our 28-year-old's lab is back. It's all-normal, and the pregnancy test is negative. Imagine that! She may have been pregnant once, but not today. When I talk to her again, she relates that the bleeding had been much worse roughly two weeks ago. She further relates that she's had no spotting or cramping in the last day. I suggest that if she does not want to get pregnant that she needs to be more conscientious about birth control. It is difficult to tell whether she is happy or sad about the news. I send her on her way with suggested follow-up. She is Rh positive and thus does not need RhoGAM.

In the case of spontaneous and completed abortions, it's important to know the patient's Rh status. Women who are Rh negative, and have an Rh-positive fetus, need to get RhoGAM if the fetus is delivered or even aborted. If this is not done, the mother can develop antibodies to the Rh-positive blood of the fetus. On subsequent pregnancies, this can produce a complication known as hydrops fetalis where the fetus is killed by the mother's immune system. RhoGAM is an immunoglobulin preparation that prevents the mother from becoming sensitized to Rh-positive fetal blood. It works by binding to the fetal blood and allowing the mother's immune system to clear it away, without her needing to form her own antibodies to the fetal blood.

My next patient is a 55-year-old morbidly obese white female who slipped on the ice on her porch and landing on her buttocks. She complains of pain in her lower back and tailbone. I give her some Toradol (an anti-inflammatory) and send her off for x-ray.

6:00 PM

In the meantime, see an 11-year-old white male who had fallen roller skating yesterday and is complaining of wrist pain. He follows our 55-year-old down to Radiology.

While this is being done, I see a 7-year-old white female with fever and cough. Today she's been coughing so hard that she gags herself and vomits. Her exam is unremarkable, but I do an influenza screen for good measure.

Our 55-year-old and our 11-year-old return from Radiology at about the same time. All their films are normal. The woman is given something for discomfort, and the boy is given an ace wrap. They're both sent on their way with routine instructions.

The influenza screen on our 11-year-old is negative. He's just got a bad cold. I give him a stronger cough medicine and send him on his way.

Then we move into the category of foolish adolescents. It's a 15-year-old white male who got mad at his parents and punched out a wall. He's having a lot of pain and swelling in his hand. No doubt! He's lucked out and hasn't broken anything. Ice and an anti-inflammatory will speed his recovery. I spend some time counseling about anger management. With this kid, I doubt it will make a difference.

This type of traumatic mechanism frequently results in what's known as a boxer's fracture. This usually involves the bone at the base of the little finger. If it's not treated properly it can result in a dominant hand that does not close properly. When the object struck is another person's face there's the potential complication of knuckle lacerations. The human mouth is a relatively dirty place, and harbors a lot of nasty bacteria. This combination can lead to an incredibly bad infection of the hand and adjacent structures. It often requires open debridement and intravenous antibiotics. So for you bar room brawlers out there, take heed!

For a Sunday night, our patient load is pretty light. It must be that people don't want to brave the weather. Who knows?

I see yet another sore throat. It's an 18-year-old white male who's had a sore throat for the last day or two. He has a negative strep test, but still wants an antibiotic. No surprise there! I give him what he wants and send him on his way.

A dramatic 13-year-old white female with sharp rib pain follows this. There's been no history of trauma, but she has focal tenderness at the rib margin. I get a x-ray for good measure, and of course it's normal. This is likely musculoskeletal, and it is reasonable to treat it symptomatically. I give her something for discomfort and send her on her way.

Next is a 2-year-old white male who had a tonsillectomy the day before yesterday. The mother states that he just won't eat or drink. She has giving nothing for discomfort as she says the kid "just spits it out." She's sure he's dehydrated despite the fact that he's had 3 or 4 wet diapers today. On exam, his hydration status is excellent, and I relate this to the mother. I suggest that she try Tylenol suppositories overnight, commenting that it's pretty hard for him to spit them out. She can check in with his surgeon in the morning. It's improbable that he could become dehydrated between now and then.

My last patient for the evening is an 88-year-old white female who's fallen at the nursing home. She complains of pain all long her left side. She is demented and pleasantly confused. Using my best Veterinary Medicine, I x-ray everything that seems to hurt. Except for some arthritic changes, the films are normal. I send her back to the nursing home with the suggestion that they use her Darvocet (a mild pain medicine) as necessary.

The remaining two hours of my shift were completely uneventful. My relief arrives and I head out the door. I note perhaps half a dozen people coming into the lobby as I make my way towards my car. It's not my problem!

12:00 AM

Shift 7

"Pioneering the limits of human endurance! "

Saturday—18 Hours

4:15 AM

Today is going to be a really bad day. I've just spent the night puking my guts out, and all I have to look forward to is two back-to-back 18-hour shifts in the ER. Oh joy!

This is one of the drawbacks of working with a small group. Getting sick is just not an option. I called the doctor on duty to let him know that I might be a little late. I made some other calls to see if I could arrange coverage for a while, but I didn't have much luck. I vomited, hopefully one last time, and crawled into my Honda, bucket in lap, and headed on down the road. I live well over an hour from where I work, and today the ride is exceedingly unpleasant.

5:30 PM

Immediately upon my arrival, the doctor on duty is ready to bolt. He has little sympathy for my plight. I'm sure it's a problem he's faced himself. All well, that's why they call me Superman. The deck has just been cleared, but I'm sure that will change shortly.

No sooner do I have the thought, than the first squad of the day arrives. It's a 95-year-old white female from a local nursing home with progressive shortness of breath. She has a presumed pneumonia, and has been on antibiotics, breathing treatments, and oxygen for the last several days. Despite this, she's getting progressively worse, and her oxygen saturation keeps dropping. My immediate gestalt is that she's on deaths doorstep. Luckily, she comes with that magic piece of paper, her advance directives, which list her as a DNR. This makes my job quite a bit easier. Without this piece of paper, we'd be putting her on a ventilator. It seems apparent that more than just pneumonia is going on. I order a full cardiac work-up, including arterial blood gases (the gold standard for measuring blood oxygen). Every way I look at it, despite maximum supplemental oxygen, oxygen delivery to her tissue really sucks. I have the respiratory therapist do additional breathing treatments, and I empirically give her both Morphine (the narcotic that can rapidly improve heart failure) and Lasix (a diuretic). Several minutes later, her chest x-ray reveals both a bilateral pneumonia as well as significant congestive heart failure.

While maximum medical management is in progress on this patient, I zip over to see the other "emergency" that has arrived. It's a 65-year-old white female who's felt dizzy for the last two hours. She's had this multiple times in the past, and it's been attributed to a viral inner ear infection. Previously, it was treated symptomatically and resolved. Rather than wait an hour-and-a-half and see her regular doctor, or call her regular doctor and have a script called in, she chooses to come to the emergency room. She wants to start treatment immediately "before it gets worse." Fine! Of course, her exam is benign. I put her on some Antivert (a dizziness medicine) and kick her out the door.

There isn't a lot more to add our 95-year-old. I'm not going to fix her here in the Emergency Room. I call the doctor covering for her regular physician, and get her shipped upstairs to the ICU.

It seems to be turning into a geriatric Saturday! On the scanner I hear the squads out on a 99-year-old with chest pain. Less than 10 minutes later they encode and are inbound with the patient.

It's a 99-year-old white male, who lives alone, and has been having early morning chest pain for the last several days. It's getting progressively worse. He was given nitroglycerine by the paramedics and the squad, and is pretty much symptom free on arrival. His EKG has new changes, and suggests that something's going on with his heart. Despite his current lack of symptoms, I give him the full range of heart protective medicines. This includes Aspirin, oxygen, Lopressor, nitroglycerine paste, and Lovenox. These are all medicines that we've talked about previously. I order routine cardiac laboratory. The patient does have slightly elevated heart enzymes, so has likely had a small heart attack. He doesn't, however, meet the criteria for TPA (the clot buster drug). I contact his doctor, and he's shipped up to the ICU for further care.

All through this time I'm trying very hard to keep from tossing my cookies, given my own ongoing illness. Thankfully, up to now most of my patients have been sicker than I am. This is almost an unusual eventuality. I get a brief respite at this point, and wander back to my call room to try and catnap.

Zzzz...

8:00 AM

My wake-up call is a 5-year-old black male who's had a cough overnight. He's in absolutely no distress, but he does have a noticeable cough. He has a label of "asthma," but is on no asthma medications. When I listen to his chest, it's very wheezy. His mother is convinced that he has pneumonia, and is sure he needs to be admitted to the hospital. I scratch my head. His oxygen level is 100%, and I do a chest x-ray that is completely normal. I have our respiratory therapist give him a breathing treatment, which cures both his wheezing and his cough.

The most common presentation of exacerbation of asthma in an asthmatic is nighttime cough. This kid fits the bill nicely. It can be triggered by most anything, including viral upper respiratory infections.

With some difficulty, I convince the mother that her child's going to be fine. I put him back on breathing treatments, and cover him with steroids and an antibiotic (for good measure). This is pretty well maximum treatment for exacerbation of asthma, and is perhaps more aggressive than is really needed for this child. With pediatric cases, it's frequently more about treating the parent than treating the child. I try to feel out the parents and meet their expectations, as long as it does no harm.

Then we're back to geriatrics. It's another 90-year-old white female with hip and back pain since a fall yesterday. Her regular doctor saw her, and films of her lower back were done. These were normal. She was started on a mild pain medicine for the discomfort, was unable to sleep tonight because of the pain, and presents to the Emergency Room for re-evaluation. Her exam is unremarkable. I give her the barest whiff of Nubain (an injected non-narcotic pain medicine), and send her down for some more radiation therapy (x-rays). Since she has pain in her hip as well, I also go ahead and film that hip. She is whisked down to Radiology, and apparently lost down there for couple hours.

Meanwhile, another squad is inbound. It seems that they no more than encode than they're at our door. It's an 85-year-old white male, with known advanced lung disease from smoking, whose had progressive shortness of breath through the morning. He's working pretty hard to breathe, and when I listen to his chest, he has little air movement. I have my respiratory therapist start stacking breathing treatments, and my nurse gives him some intravenous Solu-Medrol (a steroid). I get routine cardiac laboratory as well as arterial blood gases. I note that he has a fever, so I get a set of blood cultures as well.

The respiratory crisis associated with advanced lung disease from smoking, COPD (chronic obstructive pulmonary disease), usually has a significant asthmatic component. Much of the treatment is very similar to the treatment of asthmatics. This involves the use of breathing medicine (Ventolin, Atrovent), steroids, and oxygen.

COPD is a combination of asthma, chronic bronchitis, and emphysema. The asthma is due to spasm of the airways that's associated with inflammation. The chronic bronchitis is due to chronic irritation and chronic inflammation, with subsequent mucous production, leading to chronic sputum production. The emphysema is due to progressive destruction and coalescence of the small air sacs within the lung, secondary to the toxic effects of cigarette smoke.

In our 85-year-old, we seem to be making some headway by our objective numbers, but clinically he's not looking a lot better. His arterial blood gases show that he is holding onto significant amounts of carbon dioxide. Carbon dioxide makes the blood more acidic and makes the patient feel more short of breath. If it's high enough, it can produce what's known as carbon dioxide narcosis. The elevated carbon dioxide is usually due to the respiratory rate being inadequate to allow for its exchange. If carbon dioxide narcosis progresses far enough, the patient will become comatose, his respiratory rate will drop further, his carbon dioxide level will increase further, his oxygen level will drop, and he will die.

This is a point where some counterintuitive physiology comes into play. Folks with advanced lung disease often have a very disordered physiology. In the normal folks, respiratory drive is driven first by elevation in carbon dioxide, and secondly by decreases in oxygen. In a person with COPD, the carbon dioxide mechanism is often lost, and the respiratory drive comes strictly from decreases in oxygen level. Under normal circumstances, this is not a big problem. However, when a person with COPD gets in trouble, this is where it becomes an issue. The COPD patient has little pulmonary reserve. Respiratory illness, even the common cold, can tip them over the edge so that they become more hypoxic (their oxygen levels drops). At this point, they are frequently put on supplemental oxygen. This is where it becomes counterintuitive. If they are given "too much oxygen" it can fool the hypoxic drive into thinking that the crisis is over. The respiratory rate then drops, carbon dioxide climbs, and oxygen levels plummet despite there being increased oxygen available. It becomes a matter of subtle adjustments in supplemental oxygen to ensure the patient gets enough additional oxygen without getting too much. Of course, if you get behind the power curve and the patient becomes comatose, about the only way to recover is to put the patient on a ventilator.

Our 85-year-old is facing just this problem. He really needs to be on a ventilator if are going to optimize treatment. In discussion with the family, this is not an option. The patient has previously voiced that he does not want to be on a ventilator, nor does he want any aggressive resuscitation done should his condition worsened. Given the severity of his underlying disease, and his advanced age, this is reasonable.

By this time, a lot of the objective data is back. The patient has a good size pneumonia. I spent time tweaking his oxygen, and start some intravenous antibiotics. I contact his regular doctor and arrange for admission to the hospital.

About this time, our 90-year-old, with back and hip pain, finally makes it back from the Radiology Department. Her x-rays look like the x-rays of a 90-year-old, and there is no evidence of any bony injury. She is sleeping comfortably, and feeling no pain. I adjust her pain medicines, increase the arthritis medicine that she's already on, talk the case over with the family, and send her away.

Meanwhile, more worried well are filtering in. Next is a 32-year-old white male who 10 minutes before had slipped and fallen on the ice. He is complaining of some rib pain. We get him filmed, and of course they're normal. The real agenda is that he wants to get out of work. As I commented before, I sometimes feel we should just leave work release forms in the lobby. This would save us from doing significant amounts of unnecessary testing, and would dramatically reduce our paperwork.

I also see a 3-year-old white female who was sent over from the doctor's office to have a forehead laceration repaired with Dermabond (skin glue). The family was under the impression that this will produce a better cosmetic appearance. In reality, the outcome is about the same as long as the glue is applied and cared for correctly. I give them what they want, and send them on their way.

We seem to have another lull, and so I head back to my call room to try for another nap.

Zzzz...

I managed about an hour before the next crisis rolls in. It's a 65-year-old white female who slipped a home and wound up doing the splits. She's now having some thigh pain. Of course she's tried nothing for this. She's obviously pulled some muscles in her thighs. I put her on an anti-inflammatory, and give her a few pain pills for good measure.

We then get a very unusual case. It's a 35-year-old white female who is brought in by squad in with involuntary twitching. She has a long psychiatric history, which sets off the alarm bells in my head. She is thrashing about on the cot, but is completely awake and alert. She's hyperventilating to beat the band, and is having some tetanic muscle contractions due to this. Unfortunately, I can't blame all her symptoms on the hyperventilation. She had just started a new arthritis medicine that morning, and the side effect profile of the drug does include tremors and muscle spasms. It turns out she had this happen in the past, and they were unable to find the cause. Previously, the symptoms resolve spontaneously. Just for grins, I give her a fair sized dose of Ativan (a tranquilizer). Several minutes later, she is cured. In the end, who knows? I recommend that she discontinues the arthritis medicine, and check in with her regular physician at the first of the week.

12:00 PM

The cafeteria food looks really bad. Luckily, I've brought along some bagels, so I have one of these.

The doctors' offices are now closed, so now the fun begins.

The first of the new crew of afternoon patients is a 5-year-old white female with right ear pain and drainage for the last two to three days. Why she couldn't have been seen in the office before this time, who knows? She has a red eardrum and pus in her ear canal. This qualifies as both an otitis media and an otitis externa. This just means that there is infection on both sides of the eardrum. She's put on an oral antibiotic as well as an antibiotic eardrop. She can follow-up in a week to 10 days.

Next is a 42-year-old white male, a road warrior and patient of doctor NONE, who works at UNEM, and is insured by SELF. He's getting to be quite a frequent flier, and usually comes in quite drunk. He tells me that he struck his wrist on a car door several days ago and that it hurts. Surprisingly enough, he actually appears sober today. I film his wrist and he does have a small fracture, although it is more consistent with a boxing injury. I put on a split and suggest that he follow-up with local orthopedic doctors. He probably won't, but there's not much I can do about that.

A 6-year-old black female with a fever, sore throat, runny nose, and cough follows this. She does appear to have a ear infection, otherwise it seems like a cold. I do a strep test that is negative, and start her on some Amoxicillin (an antibiotic) for her ear infection.

My next patient is a bloody mess. It's a 90-year-old white female who bumped her shin trying to get into an SUV. She split it open, and then proceeded to bleed all over everything. It's a pretty impressive wound for the mechanism, but the elderly often have very thin skin that's easily torn. I spend about half an hour putting her leg back together, and send her on her way.

The dueling toes follow this. Two unrelated patients, a 22-year-old white female and a 55-year-old white male both managed to stub their little toe. X-rays are done, and the younger of the two is normal, while the older has a fracture. The fractured toe is taped to the one next door, and both patients were sent on their way.

I see a 21-year-old white male with three days of cold symptoms. He wants to be on an antibiotic, so I oblige. Surprisingly enough (Not!), he wants a work release as well. Again, in the spirit of McMedicine, I give him what he wants.

The afternoon is going rather slowly. We seem to be getting a patient every 30 to 40 minutes. When shifts are like this, you feel like you're in the eye of a storm, and that all hell is about to break loose at any minute. As we near the evening mealtime, this prophecy is likely to come true. I don't know what is about mealtimes, but they tend to be very busy.

We return to pediatrics for a while, with a 15-month-old white male who fell on a toy at home and managed a forehead laceration. This is Dermabonded (skin glue).

6:00 PM

The evening selection at the cafeteria is every bit as bad as lunch. It's a good thing I have a lot of bagels along.

I see a 35-year-old obese white female with a painful red area in her armpit. She appears to have nicked herself shaving, and now has a local skin infection in the area. I put her on an appropriate antibiotic, and send her on her way.

This is followed immediately by a 2-year-old white male who fell while playing at home and bumped his head. There was no loss of consciousness, and the child has been appropriate since. He was brought in because he has a small lump on his head. What ever happened to the days when people had common sense?

My next case becomes somewhat interesting. It's a 65-year-old white male, a diabetic with severe diabetic neuropathy (he has little sensation in his feet). It seems that his wife noted a hole in his foot, and insisted he have it looked at. I do a x-ray of his foot, and find that he has a needle embedded in his heel. On x-ray, it looks to be immediately below the surface of the skin, but when I try to remove it with a pair of splinter forceps, I can't. Not to be outdone by a needle, I take the patient down to the Radiology suite and use fluoroscopy to grab the needle and jerk it out. I put him on an antibiotic for good measure, and recommend that he has it looked at again at the first of the week.

No weekend seems complete without an assortment of fruits and nuts. Next is a 33-year-old white male who definitely falls into the fruit and nut category. He has what we refer to as a "globally positive review of systems." What this means is that any symptom you might think up this patient says he has. Of course that makes it very difficult to figure out just what's going on. In the end, I get it narrowed down to cold symptoms and diarrhea. The patient is convinced that he's dehydrated. He insists that he's lost 25 lbs. in the last 24 hours. Now of course, the only way this could happen would be if he'd cut off a leg. Since I see both of his legs are attached, I think this is improbable. I do a range of lab, and surprise, it's all normal. This complement's a normal exam. And now for the real agenda, this whole ridiculous drama is just because the patient wants a work release. Fine! McMedicine at its finest!

The next patient is another head scratcher. It's a 6-year-old white male who allegedly has a fever. At some point during the day he also had apparently said that his penis itches. In the ER, the patient has a normal temperature and denies the itching. His exam is normal, as is a urinalysis. In the end, I recommend symptomatic treatment with follow-up as necessary. Who knows?

As we move later into the evening, we start to see those folks who injured themselves earlier in the day. As bedtime approaches, they feel that it needs looking after. The next patient is a case in point. It's a 17-year-old white male who had fallen skating this morning and is complaining of a painful wrist. A x-ray is done which demonstrates a small fracture in his wrist known as a torus, or buckle, fracture. In the short term, this just warrants a splint. I have it applied and recommend that he follows up first the week.

Oh, I've forgotten to mention the progress of my own affliction. Along about noon my stomach finally calmed down, and I began feeling mostly normal (or at least as normal as someone can feel who hasn't slept for 36 hours). All well, C'est La Vie.

And we're back to the fruits and nuts in the form of a 55-year-old white female who comes in by squad with police in tow. It seems she's tired of life, and took a handful of pain pills in an apparent attempt to end her life. A family member immediately called 911, and the rest is history. She's not very talkative. It seems she's taken perhaps 20 or 30 Vicodin. This is a combination of Tylenol and Hydrocodone (a mild narcotic). Of the two ingredients, the Tylenol poses the greater risk. Poison Control is contacted, and as expected, they recommend lavaging the patient's stomach, instilling activated charcoal, and getting drug levels. If warranted, a Tylenol "antidote" called Mucomyst can be used to help prevent Tylenol associated liver failure. I get this patient started, and then go look after the other patients that have checked in.

There is a 2-year-old Hispanic male with painful urination that I have the nurse get a urinalysis on. There's also a 2-year-old Hispanic female with fever, cough, and sore throat that I have the nurse get an influenza screen and strep screen on.

Luckily the witching hour is approaching, and my relief shows up early. I am dead tired with a capital "D." I check my patients out to the next shift, grab some blankets, and head upstairs to the hospital floor to find an empty room. This quickly done, I am, as the saying goes, "out like a light." And none soon...

12:00 AM

Zzzz...

Shift 8

"No end in sight..."

Sunday—18 Hours

6:00 AM

It's amazing what a few hours of sleep can do for your disposition. I actually feel like a human being again. Surprisingly, yesterday was slow enough that I was able to keep up with my dictation. This is the first time in weeks that I haven't started Sunday morning with 30 or 40 charts to finish. It seems a rare luxury. But all good things come to an end, and no good deed goes unpunished. Usually, when we have a good Saturday, Sunday is hell. Let the floodgates open!

My first patient of the day is a 72-year-old white male with back and thigh pain. It seems he twisted his back getting out of his truck yesterday. Of course, he's tried nothing for this. His exam is normal. There was no specific trauma. I put him on Daypro (an anti-inflammatory), and Vicodin (a mild narcotic), and send him on his way.

After a short reprieve, I see a 40-year-old white male with cold symptoms. He's smoked two packs a day for the better part of 30 years, and seems unable to accept that there might be some association between his chronic recurrent respiratory illness and his smoking. He wants to be back on an antibiotic, so I go ahead and oblige.

9:00 AM

Amazingly, we have almost two hours with no one in the department. Then I see an 11-year-old white male with "swelling of his choo-choo." Hmmm...Well it seems that he had been swimming in a heavily chlorinated pool the night before, and shortly thereafter developed some edema (soft tissue swelling) of the foreskin of his penis. It really isn't bothering him. It just looks strange. Of course, this is likely either an allergic reaction or skin irritation due to the chemical compounds used in the pool. It's likely that it would get better even if nothing was done, but people come to the Emergency Room for a cure. I put him on a few days of Prednisone (a steroid) and Vistaril (an antihistamine). Though this is overkill, it should get the job done.

Then it's time for the squads to start rolling in, and our first one is a 90-year-old white female who had taken a fall the night before. She couldn't get up, and had spent the night on the floor. She's feeling no pain, but states that she, "just feels weak." It seems this weakness has been coming on for the last several days. She is in a new atrial fibrillation (a heart arrhythmia) with a heart rate in the 180's to 190's. This by itself could make a 90-year-old very weak. When the heart beats this fast at rest, it doesn't empty properly. The end result can be a heart that functions at as little as 25% of normal capacity. One question to ask is, "why does this patient have this arrhythmia?" I start a cardiac work up to look for the answer.

In the meantime, I see a 35-year-old white female with two hours of calf pain. The more I talked to her, the more I find myself attaching a label of hypochondriac. It seems she's scheduled for elective surgery next week, and at her preoperative physical exam had been asked about calf pain. This morning one calf seemed sore. She looked up sore calves in her home medical book, and is now convinced that she has a blood clot in her leg. She has no risk factors for blood clots, but she's not going to be satisfied until I ultrasound leg and prove that it's normal. I send her off to ultrasound for our McMedicine best.

By this time I begin getting information back on our weak 90-year-old. I have been trying to slow her heart rate down with a beta-blocker, Lopressor. This has met with some success. I see that her heart enzymes are elevated, so it's likely she's working on a small heart attack. This easily accounts for the atrial fibrillation. I contact her doctor and make arrangements to get her out of my department.

A while later, my hypochondriac returns from ultrasound. Of course, it's completely normal, as expected. I provide some reassurance, and empirically put her on an anti-inflammatory.

One of the real problems with all the health information that's widely available to the lay public is that they have no means of putting it in context. They can look up which symptoms are associated with any given disease, but they have no way to determine how probable it is that they may have this disease. Any given symptom may be present in 50 or 60 diseases. Of course, the natural tendency of the layperson is to fixate on the absolute worst disease. If one were to rank-order diseases by increasing probability that a specific person would have a specific disease, frequently the most probable affliction is the most benign. In an otherwise healthy, 35-year-old white female, this is definitely the case. This is also why I know in advance, with greater than 99% certainty, that this patient is going to have a normal ultrasound.

Our next crisis of the day is a 50-year-old white female who felt a "crunch" in her knee last night, and is having increasing pain. There was no trauma, and she has taken nothing for the discomfort. Of course, her knee films are fine. Any number of things can produce a crunch, but they are all initially treated pretty much the same. I put her on some Daypro (an anti-inflammatory) and some Vicodin (a mild narcotic). She can use crutches for now, and follow-up is it just doesn't get better. There are few spontaneous injuries in a person like this. She's probably just managed to sprain it. I head her towards the door.

A 75-year-old white female who accidentally struck her hand on the car door follows this. She's concerned that it's swollen so much. Her films are normal, but the back of her hand is pretty good size. She's likely ruptured one of the small blood vessels back there and has a hematoma. This is treated symptomatically, and resolves over a week or two.

I also see a 40-year-old white female with several days of neck pain, sore throat, and difficulty swallowing. She has a history of a thyroid tumor that required surgical excision of the majority of her thyroid. She does have a nodule in her neck, as well as multiple enlarged lymph nodes. She also has significant enlargement of her tonsils on one side.

In this patient, there are two potential issues to consider. First, there is the possibility of a peritonsillar abscess (a collection of pus under the tonsil that requires surgical drainage), and second there is the more remote possibility of a neck mass, possibly a malignancy. I do routine lab, and send her off for a CT scan of her neck. That will put it to rest one way or the other.

While she is off at Radiology, I see a 12-year-old white female with fever, sore throat, and cough. The nurse has done a strep test that is positive. I put her on some Amoxicillin (an antibiotic) and send her off.

There is also a 19-year-old white female with nausea and body aches. She is sure she's pregnant. She's a couple months overdue for her Depo-Provera shot (a 3-month birth control shot), is still sexually active, and is using no other form of birth control. She wants a pregnancy test. Now how this is going to change things today, or this weekend, I don't know. It's a pretty expensive way to get a pregnancy test, but whatever! I have it done. I doubt she's paying for it anyway.

The lab on our 40-year-old makes it back about the same time as the patient returns from Radiology. The CT was normal, but she does have a positive strep test. I put her on some Amoxicillin (an antibiotic) and recommend that she follow-up with the ENT folks about the neck nodule.

Our 19-year-old isn't pregnant, so she's probably got a mild case of the stomach bug that's making the rounds. I strongly encourage her to be more conscientious about birth control issues if she doesn't want to get pregnant. Who knows how much sunk in?

12:00 PM

Alright, time for the afternoon rush, and a rush it is.

First is a 8-year-old white male who's had a sore throat for the last couple of days. Then, earlier today, he had fallen with a straw in his mouth and cut the back of his throat. I do a strep test and it's negative. There's a superficial abrasion of the soft palate on examination. It will heal on its own and only needs symptomatic treatment.

Second is a 41-year-old white male who slipped while using a hand saw and cut his hand. It's pretty superficial, but does require a handful of stitches.

Third is a 90-year-old white male with a huge facial mass. It's been present a couple of weeks, but today a family member drags him in. It's draining some pus from one corner. This is likely an abscess, but could be a tumor that lost its blood supply, necrosed, and became infected. Whatever, its way too big for me to go near. This is one for the facial surgeon to address, so I call him, and he takes it off my hands.

Forth is a 45-year-old white male, with a known history of seizure disorder, who had a breakthrough seizure at work. I check his seizure medicine levels, and they are a little on the low side. I'm about ready to release him, when he has another seizure. I give additional meds in the department and decide to watch him for a while longer.

Fifth is an interesting case that is frequently missed by primary care doctors. It's an 85-year-old white male with several weeks of shoulder pain. His regular doctor has put him on some Vioxx (a newer arthritis medicine), but it just isn't helping. He couldn't sleep at all last night because of the increasing pain, so he winds up in my department. When I question him further, he has had increasing pain in both of his thighs as well.

The nurse tries to make an argument for atypical cardiac pain, and I do a cardiac profile just for good measure. However, that's not what's going on. The telling test to cinch the diagnosis is an ESR (Erythrocyte Sedimentation Rate). This is a measure of inflammation.

This patient, in my book, has PMR (Polymyalgia Rheumatica) until proven otherwise. The hallmark of PMR is progressive proximal muscle pain. This is a rheumatology disorder that, aside from pain, is usually benign, except for one association. PMR can be associated with temporal arteritis. This is an inflammatory disorder of arteries in the head that can have associated eye and temple pain. If untreated, it can lead to blindness and stroke. Both of these disorders are treated with steroids, often with dramatic improvement within hours.

When the lab and such is done, bingo, the ESR is significantly elevated and consistent with PMR. I start him on high dose steroids. He can follow-up with his regular doctor tomorrow.

Sixth is a 42-year-old white female with chronic ankle pain who says she's out of pain meds. She does have quite a history of drug seeking. I'm feeling generous though, and get her enough to get by until the morning. From there she can negotiate with her regular doctor.

Something I'm always a bit worried about with the drug seeking, drug-abusing crowd is that some are very sneaky. Often they'll take any medicine you give, as long as the prescription has your DEA (Drug Enforcement Agency) number on it. Once they get your number (it's required on any prescription for a controlled substance), they can make more authentic appearing prescription forgeries. Once or twice a year the police come in with scripts I have allegedly written, for quantities of medicines I would never prescribe.

Seventh is an 85-year-old white male with a plugged feeding tube. He's got some problem with his esophagus and can't swallow. We can't get it opened up, so we wind up having the surgeon come in and replace it.

Eighth is a 24-year-old white male who lost control of his 4 wheeler and flipped it. He's complaining of upper chest pain. His film is suspicious for a clavicle fracture. He's put in a clavicle splint, and advised to follow-up.

Ninth is a 4-year-old white female with chicken pox. Why is this in the ER? This isn't exactly rocket science! This is treated symptomatically, and gets better on its own in 10-14 days. It can be prevented with an immunization. It seems a lot of folks still don't know this, or they have some misconceptions about its effectiveness.

Tenth is a 22-year-old white male who fell snow boarding this morning, and is complaining of shoulder pain. There is obvious deformity on the top of the shoulder. The x-ray shows a separated acromio-clavicular joint (the attachment of the clavicle to the top of the shoulder). I'm thankful that it isn't a shoulder dislocation. That is more complicated to take care of, and I'm not feeling very motivated right now. I put him in a sling with orthopedic follow-up.

Eleventh is a 20-year-old white female who had a nosebleed. She HAD one, but it has since stopped. So now she comes to the ER. She acts like she's about ready to die. When I look up in her nose, there is a small, irritated, area on the septum. I use silver nitrate to cauterize the area, just for good measure. I get a blood count that is normal. We "watch" her for an hour or so to make sure there's no other bleeding, and then send her on her way.

Oh yes, our seizure person. He had yet another seizure, despite the additional seizure medicine. He gets to spend the night.

The twelfth is somewhat more impressive. It's a 36-year-old white male with about a half-hour history of sudden onset flank pain. He's sweating bullets, and rolling around on the cart like there's a dagger protruding from his side. Now this is what a kidney stone looks like. He's not able to get us any urine for urinalysis, but in the end, I send him off for IVP (intravenous pyelogram, a special x-ray of the kidneys and their collecting system). This guy is completely obstructed on that side by a kidney stone. It takes quite a bit of intravenous Demerol (a big-gun narcotic) to get him comfortable. I chat with his doctor and the urologist, and we get him admitted.

Thirteenth is a 40-year-old white male, yet another smoker, with cough and congestion. He doesn't want to hear about his smoking. His exam is fine. He wants an antibiotic, fine! He would likely get better quicker if he threw away the cigarettes.

6:00 PM

Fourteenth is a 41-year-old white male who slipped on the ice and has ankle pain. The film tells the story and it's broken in two places. This needs a surgery, so the orthopedic doctor is called to take over.

Fifteenth is a 38-year-old white female with abdominal cramping. She'd had a laparoscopy ("Band-Aid" surgery done with a fiber optic scope) for adhesions (scarring in the abdomen that produces pain) earlier in the week, and has been on Tylenol with codeine since. When all is said and done, she's constipated from the codeine. She doesn't want an enema, so I send her home with a laxative. She'll live.

Sixteenth is a 22-year-old white male with a sore throat for a day. The nurse has gone ahead and gotten a strep screen, and it's positive. I put him on some Amoxicillin (an antibiotic) and out the door.

Seventeenth is a 30-year-old white male with ear pain. Surprisingly, he's got an ear infection, and he also is put on Amoxicillin. Ear infections are relatively uncommon in adults.

Eighteenth is an 18-year-old white female, also with ear pain, who also has an ear infection, and gets Amoxicillin. This is getting monotonous. It's also breaking the laws of statistical averages.

Nineteenth is a 15-year-old white male who got pissed off and punched out a window. He cut up his hand quite a bit. It takes some talking to get him to let me repair it, but I finally manage.

Twentieth is a 6-year-old Hispanic female with fever, sore throat, and vomiting for the day. She's smiling up at me and in no distress. Her strep test is negative, so she's likely got one of the stomach bugs. I give her mother some Phenergan suppositories (an anti-nausea medicine) to have available, and send her on.

Twenty-first is a 32-year-old white female who's 8 weeks pregnant. She's been having abdominal cramping and vaginal bleeding. Her ultrasound shows a nonviable fetal sac that appears about ready to be expelled. In the end she opts to go home to let nature take its course.

And my replacement is here, so I am out of here.

12:00 AM

Shift 9

"Life and death…"

Wednesday—18 Hours

12:00 PM

It's been a while since I've worked a weekday shift. This is an overnight, and that's not exactly my favorite.

I've been left a 45-year-old white male, now in Radiology, who had several pallets fall on him at work. It sounds like he may have been knocked out, and he's also complaining of low back pain. He's off getting a head CT, neck films, a chest film, and back films.

In the mean time I see a 14-month-old white female who had gotten into a bottle of Zyrtec (an antihistamine) that was sitting on the counter at home. It is uncertain how much the little kiddo may have ingested, if any. Of course the kid's doing just fine when we start, but that doesn't last for long. Poison Control recommends we lavage and charcoal the kid. The girl is decidedly unhappy with having a tube shoved down her nose and into her stomach, but we get it done. The stomach is washed out, and the charcoal is shot in. We watch the kid for a couple of hours before sending her home. The mom really doesn't connect that it was her fault that the child had to endure all of this. After all, she was the one that left the medicine out. Ah well…

I also see a 28-year-old white male, one of our local road warriors, who had punched out his buddy a week or so ago. His hand is now very much infected. These tend to be very nasty infections that can be hard to get under control. They sometimes require that the hand be flayed open and irrigated out. I call his regular doctor and he is admitted for intravenous antibiotics. I'm betting the orthopedic doctors are going to be involved before everything is done.

Well our 45-year-old finally makes it back, and it looks like he's broken his neck and his back. The back injury isn't too worrisome, it's a stable fracture and will just cause pain for a couple of months. The neck injury is a bit more worrisome. If unstable, this is how quadriplegics are made. I call the local trauma center, and make arrangements to have him evaluated there. Whenever I've got someone with a significant neck injury, it's going to be a neurosurgeon that makes the final call about what, if anything, needs to be done. He's trussed up and hauled away by squad.

Next is a 24-year-old white female who stubbed her toe a week ago. Why is this an emergency when every doctor office is open? Who knows? Her films are normal. Then she's pissed off that we won't give her samples of pain meds. Ah well…

Wow, now for a real emergency! A 90-year-old white male is being sent over from their doctor's office because he hasn't pooped in the last week. He is packed up, and now its been made our job to dig him out. Multiple enemas later, and several pounds lighter, he is on his way smiling.

Then we're back to the ridiculous and the sublime. It's a 45-year-old white female with tooth pain for a week. She won't go to the dentists because she says she doesn't have enough money. This doesn't stop her from coming to the ER daily. Charges from a single ER visit would probably be enough to get all her teeth pulled, and that's what she needs. Of course, we're not likely to get paid for all these visits she's making. She has a doctor who she's not bothered to contact. I give him a ring and make arrangement for her to get some samples of an antibiotic for a few days. That should help temporize her tooth pain for a while.

Boy we're developing a theme here. Next is a 60-year-old white male with 4-5 days of constipation that's just not responding to Milk of Magnesia. An enema from below and a laxative from above should have him spraying the walls.

6:00 PM

Hmmm. It's kind of a pud day. I've managed to get caught up on my writing.

I see a 22-year-old white female with wrist pain. There was no specific injury, but her industrial job is pretty tough on her wrists. She's recently had carpal tunnel surgery, but that's well healed. She has tenderness along several of the tendons in her forearm. She's sure she's done some mortal injury, so we get a film, and guess what? Normal! She's managed a tendonitis. It's a typical use-related injury. I put her on some Naproxen (an anti-inflammatory) and Vicodin (a mild narcotic). She can do activity as tolerated, and follow-up as needed.

As we move further into the evening hours, I'm sure business will pick up as usual. It never fails. The doctor's offices have been closed for a couple of hours, and folks are beginning to stew. We're bound to get the worried well who just can't get through the night without their doctor fix.

Sometimes people are hard to understand. I'm not sure if they think they're pulling one over on us, or just what. There are certain people that apparently wait until just after their doctor's offices closed, and then race to the Emergency Room to get something for their "headaches." Maybe it's that their doctor doesn't give them what they want, or perhaps they're just getting off work themselves (surprisingly, some of these folks do have jobs). I don't know. This even seems to happen on the weekends, after the offices close at noon. Our next patient is a case in point. It's a 35-year-old white male with his typical "migraine" for the last several days. I give him my concoction, wait a while, and send him packing.

This followed by a 32-year-old white female who complains of red mattery eyes. She was actually seen approximately 10 days ago, diagnosed with a bilateral conjunctivitis (pinkeye), and put on antibiotic eyedrops. She says she feels better, but her eyes look like shit. There is diffuse bleeding under the conjunctiva such that the whites of her eyes look like blood. She just wants more eyedrops, and she tells me she has no money for this. Now, of course, she has money for the cigarettes in her pocket.

If this is just a simple eye infection, I would expect it to be fully resolved by now. Given its persistence, I make a call to the local ophthalmologist. Eyes are nothing to mess with. If improperly managed, an eye problem can generate huge malpractice claims.

In the meantime, I see a 101-year-old white female, who still lives independently. She has no significant medical history, but has had increasing exertional shortness of breath for the last week. This lady is incredible, but despite excellent genetics, we are all going to die of something someday (hopefully not today). My impression is that she's probably had a silent heart attack in the last week or so, and has (unknowingly) been putting herself through cardiac rehabilitation. Her EKG has some subtle changes, and I order a full cardiac work-up for good measure. Lying on the cot she has no symptoms, but if she has to walk across the room, she gets winded. We'll see what we find.

The ophthalmologist makes it in, and is underwhelmed with the eye problem. He feels this is just a common, non-threatening, complication of adenovirus infection. This is the same virus that causes the common cold. It is self limited, usually resolves spontaneous within a few weeks, and only requires supportive treatment. He just recommends artificial tears. This is available inexpensively over-the-counter. Our patient will perhaps have to smoke a few less cigarettes this week.

Our latest crisis then distracts me. It's an 85-year-old white man who's had intermittent visual hallucinations for the last day. It seems he keeps seeing things that no one else can. His family seems to believe that these symptoms are because his blood pressure is too high. However, it's only slightly elevated, by no means dangerously so. In general, this guy isn't tracking very well. I'd put him in the category of "pleasantly confused." I start our routine delirium work-up to try and find something that we can fix. This includes a head scan, and a range of other tests.

In the elderly, delirium, or altered mental status, is very common. It usually represents one of the three D's of geriatrics: delirium, dementia, or major depression. In this population, these often have identical symptoms, but very different prognosis. Delirium and depression are often reversible, but dementia is not (at least not at this time). The goal is to find something we can fix. This might be something metabolic, or something infectious. Sometimes it can even be drug related. Often the elderly are on a range of pain medicines, any of which can produce confusion. Another cause that's often overlooked in this population is alcohol abuse. Significant numbers of the elderly who present to the Emergency Department have problems with chronic alcohol abuse. In this patient, we'll see.

Back to our 101-year-old, it's really looking like my thoughts are correct. Her chest x-ray shows new onset congestive heart failure, and her heart enzymes are elevated. She's also anemic, which may play a contributing role. I put her on the appropriate protective medicines, and call her regular physician to get her admitted.

My next patient is an 8-year-old white female with a 2-3 week history of intermittent abdominal pain and vomiting. When her symptoms began, everyone in the family had similar symptoms. However, they got better and she didn't. Tonight she apparently had some abdominal cramping and a single episode of vomiting. Her exam is completely normal. She appears tired, but she's in no distress. She has no focal abdominal tenderness that would be suspicious for appendicitis. Given the duration of symptom, I order range of lab and what not, in order to provide reassurance than nothing else is going on.

I also see a 30-year-old white female with a rash. This is yet another "emergency" rash and is very unimpressive. It looks like she had gotten into something she is allergic to. It is benign enough that some over-the-counter Benadryl, or even topical hydrocortisone, would be adequate. I tell her this diplomatically.

Then there is a 50-year-old obese white female who's had several episodes of vomiting through the evening. With this, she has allegedly vomited some blood. She has no other symptoms aside from some nausea and vague and upper abdominal discomfort. She probably has the stomach bug that has been going around. Her vomiting may have irritated her esophagus enough to produce a small amount of bleeding. This is fairly common, and usually benign. I order routine lab to provide reassurance that nothing else is going on, and ask the nurse to put down a nasogastric tube and verify if there's blood in her stomach. We'll see…

Back to our 85-year-old who's occasionally see'in the bugs on the walls. His head scan is normal for a 85-year-old, as is the majority of his lab. The exception is that his urinalysis shows a severe urinary tract infection. An interesting thing about bladder infections in the elderly is that they can present in unusual ways. A young person with a bladder infection may just have some pain and burning with urination. An older person may have no pain or burning, but may instead have confusion. Why is this? I'm not sure that it's well understood. The bottom line is that treating the infection usually cures the confusion (at least back to the patient's baseline). I put him on some Levaquin, and he can follow-up with his regular physician later in the week.

As for our 8-year-old, everything is normal except for her belly films. They show her to be packed with poop. This seems to be a recurring theme. She may have another little stomach bug as well, but we'll treated this pretty much the same. I give her a dose of Milk of Magnesia (a laxative) to get things moving, and some Phenergan (an anti-nausea medicine) suppositories should she need them. She needs to get plenty of fluids, and she should be fine.

Our 50-year-old has no blood in her stomach, no blood in her stools, and a normal work-up. This supports my initial impression. We can treat it symptomatically. She gets some Compazine (an anti-nausea medicine) suppositories and is sent on her way.

There's some down time prior to the next patient, so I try to get caught up on my chart dictation. I don't expect this to last for long.

And it doesn't. I then see a 12-month-old hispanic male who vomited once this evening. He's smiling, laughing, and racing around the room. I silently shake my head. Why is this kid here? Of course, his exam is completely normal. If he has anything, it's the same bug everyone else has, and warrants supportive treatment only. I try and relate this to the parents, who speak only broken English, and then get them out the door.

12:00 AM

Earlier in the evening I had been told that two patients had been triaged up to Labor and Delivery. Well, surprise, surprise, they've now been sent back down to my department.

This is one of my pet peeves about this facility. Most other places I've worked, OB patients are managed exclusively by their obstetricians. This is usually done in the Labor and Delivery Area, and the obstetrician typical checks them there. At this facility, the labor and delivery nurse checks to see if the patient is in labor, and does fetal monitoring for an hour or two. The obstetrician does not see the patient unless there is a specific obstetric problem, but the patient is then dumped back to the emergency room for further evaluation, treatment, and disposition. Personally, I think it's poor form, but that's just my opinion.

Well, tonight we've got the dueling 20-year-olds. Both are about eight months pregnant. One has a runny nose, cough, and body aches. The other has nausea, vomiting, abdominal cramping, and diarrhea. I do baseline laboratory on both, to include a blood count, electrolytes, and urinalysis. I have the nurse give intravenous fluids and an antiemetic to the puker. While waiting for the results, I try and catch a catnap.

3:00 AM

Zzzz...

4:00 AM

To no one's surprise, these girls' labs are normal. The one with the cold symptoms, I treat symptomatically. I give her something a little stronger for her body aches so she can sleep. The other, with the stomach flu symptoms, is pretty much cured with the IV. I get them both hustled out the door. And now for something really important...

4:25 AM

Zzzz...

5:00 AM

My 5:00 a.m. wakeup call is for more foolishness. There's a 35-year-old white male from one of the local manufacturing facilities with a superficial cut on his finger. This requires little more than a Band-Aid. I also have a 25-year-old white female with a toothache for an hour. I don't seem to recall going to dental school, and the dentist office opens in just a couple of hours. You'd think she could have taken Tylenol or Motrin, and made due for a couple of hours. It's not so bad that she will allow me to inject the tooth with Novocain, but apparently bad enough that she just has to have a narcotic. Fine. This is more McMedicine at its best.

Well my shift is done, and I am out of here...

6:00 AM

Shift 10

"War on the installment plan..."

Saturday—18 Hours

6:00 PM

Not much is going on when I arrive. There's an 18-year-old white male who was in a fisticuff last night after an evening of boozing. Now he's puking, and his parents are sure he has a head injury. It's more likely he has the ol "brown bottle flu." It's going to take a $1000 scan to prove it. This makes for a pretty expensive night of drinking and fighting. Ah, well. I guess it's the age-old plight of the young and stupid. We've been awaiting the results since I arrived at 6:00. It seems to be running slow in Radiology this morning.

7:00 AM

Then we're back to our usual weekend fare. It's a 30-year-old white female with her typical "migraine headache." She wants "what I got last time," which right away puts her in the frequent flyer category. At least she doesn't demand Demerol this time like she did when she was here before. I give her what she wants and she goes away.

Back to our 18-year-old. His scan is normal except a mashed nose. He may have a mild concussion, but nothing that needs anything but supportive care. He definitely has a hangover. He'll need to see an ENT doc first of the week to get his nose splinted. Otherwise, he needs to be grounded for the rest of his life.

9:00 AM

Pretty quiet till now. The squad encodes, and then almost immediately arrives. We see a 58-year-old white male who is weak and dizzy. He does have a significant history of vascular disease and hypertension. He had a large stroke in his early 50's due to a blocked artery in his neck. His exam is pretty unremarkable except for the residual of his prior stroke. He was scheduled to see his regular doctor early this morning, but felt too weak to get into his wheelchair. Who knows, I'll shotgun it and see what I uncover. I'm not optimistic that I'll uncover anything.

Meanwhile I see a 70-year-old white female with a rash since yesterday. Initially she tells me she's had no new medication or dietary changes. She then proceeds to talk my ear off about all her myriad problems. When I finally redirect her back to her burning rash, I manage to get her to tell me that she just started taking niacin, and had taken the first tablets about an hour before the symptoms started. Bingo! Niacin is notorious for producing flushing, and is the biggest reason that folks quit taking the niacin. She can take an aspirin with the niacin (this reduces the flushing), reduce the dose, split the dose, slowly taper up the dose, or stop it. She can make that decision on her own. Folks often take high dose niacin to help reduce their cholesterol. In this lady, she can't really give me a good reason why she started taking it.

While I was sequestered in the room with our red lady, a squad encodes and brings in a 21-year-old car wreck victim. She pulled out in front of another car. The roads were icy, and she was unable to stop in time. She was restrained, and there was minimal damage to the car. She's complaining of neck pain, and comes in on a backboard with a cervical collar in place. I send her off to Radiology to film her neck. It's going to be fine, but I have a medicolegal obligation to prove it.

Meanwhile, I see an 11-year-old white female who bumped her leg while playing basketball. She managed to split open her shin in the process. She's skittish as all get out, but I manage to calm her down enough to get her stitched up.

Next is a 22-year-old white female with lower abdominal pain and pain with urination. She was in just a couple of weeks ago with the same symptoms and had a significant work-up done that was normal. I start with the basics. Maybe I'll get lucky. It is noteworthy that she's 6-7 months post partum (childbirth), is sexually active, and on no birth control. She doesn't want to have any children for at least a few years. She is under the common misconception that a recent pregnancy somehow protects her from getting pregnant right away. I also hear some folks say that breast-feeding keeps you from getting pregnant. The answer to both is NOT! In a young, otherwise healthy, female you could get pregnant again as early as two weeks after delivery. Given that the baseline fertility rate in young women is roughly 85% a year, this girl is definitely tempting fate.

Back to our motor vehicle accident. Of course the films are normal. She'll live. She's out of here.

12:00 PM

Next is a 26-year-old white male with upper and lower abdominal pain for the last 3-4 days. It's helped with a 12 pack of brewskies, if that says anything to you. What a winner! I start the work-up. We'll see.

Almost immediately following is a 18-year-old obese white female, a patient of doctor NONE, with three days of fever, nausea, and vomiting. She's had a nonproductive cough as well. She's been unable to keep much of anything down. I'll give her some intravenous fluids, Toradol (an anti-inflammatory), and Compazine (an antiemetic). We'll do some baseline lab, including influenza screen, and see what we come up with.

Back to our 26-year-old. The lab is normal. He's off getting belly films. I just really doubt I'll find anything. We'll keep on plugging along.

Our 18-year-old has influenza. She didn't have her flu shot this year. With the fluids and whatnot, she's feeling much better. Now she'll hopefully remember next year to get immunized. I get her out the door with some Compazine suppositories. She can follow-up as needed.

I can't find a thing wrong with our 26-year-old. Our whole belly pain evaluation is normal. This is likely more muscular in nature. There also appears to be a component of secondary gain as he wants a work release. I'll put him on some Naproxen (an anti-inflammatory) and Ultram (a non-narcotic pain medicine). He can follow-up as needed.

We have a squad encoding. It's a little grandma from the local nursing home with left-sided abdominal pain. How exciting...

Meanwhile, I see a 14-year-old white female who fell on the ice and is having wrist and elbow pain. She's whisked off to Radiology.

And our squad patient is a 85-year-old white female with side pain since yesterday.

And another squad is encoding with an 85-year-old white male with hip pain. He's in from the nursing home after having fallen.

We also have a 17-year-old white male who fell on the ice and has low back pain. He's got a hematoma back there (a collection of blood under the skin). He likely broke a blood vessel under the skin in the fall. This is treated symptomatically, and will get better on its own in a week or two.

The 14-year-old is just bruised and sprained. Her films are fine. We'll treat her symptomatically. Her mom wants a sling for her. Fine! McMedicine is in force.

Our 85-year-old white male with the fall has normal films. He's likely just bruised himself. He is so demented that it's hard to tell if he's having any discomfort, or just what. I give him some Darvocet (Tylenol and propoxyphene) and send him back to the home.

All of the lab on our 85-year-old white female with the flank pain is normal. Now, she's had shingles at the same location in the past. She's likely got a case of post-herpetic neuralgia. This is recurrent pain that can occur in folks who have previously had shingles.

I've talked about shingles previously. It's the reactivation of chicken pox. It resides in the nerves, and can express itself at any time. It's more common in the elderly. It's treated symptomatically. I put her on some Darvocet (a mild narcotic pain medicine), and sent her on her way.

Well, the afternoon is dragging on. I'm over half way through my shift, and we're way below our usual numbers. I've been able to keep up with my chart dictation, which is unusual for a Saturday. Ah well, its feast or famine. I'm sure it'll pick up later in the day.

We apparently had about 4 inches of snow yesterday, and it was really slick. I'm glad I wasn't working then.

I'm in a marathon stretch. I work five of the next six days. Then, thankfully, I'm off for a week to Disney World.

Well, we're approaching the evening mealtime and the floodgates are opening.

First is a 29-year-old white female. She's a nonsmoking asthmatic and has had shortness of breath with chest discomfort through the morning. She's convinced she has pneumonia, and so I'm obligated to x-ray her chest to prove it's normal. I give her a breathing treatment with peak flows before and after.

Peak flows measure a person's ability to move air. You blow through a plastic contraption, and it gives you a number. There are standardized tables of what folks peak flows should be as well as what they are when a person is having trouble. It's a simple way to measure asthma severity.

This lady is blowing about half what she should be able to, and so she does have a moderate asthma exacerbation in progress. There is about a 20% improvement after a breathing treatment. She should be helped with scheduled breathing treatments. I put her on some steroid, and an inhaler, then send her on her way.

From this, we are back to another persons who's working hard to be a frequent flyer. It's a 39-year-old white female with a "migraine." She was in just last night with the same symptoms. I repeat what she'd gotten previously, but make sure she knows that it is not an option to keep coming back to the ER for this. I give her something new to try at home.

Next is real foolishness. It's a 14-year-old white male who was riding a 4-wheeler without a helmet. He stopped suddenly and slammed his face into the handlebars. This split open his jaw. He's not very happy with the thought of the repair job coming up. First though, I send him to Radiology to film his jaw.

6:00 PM

In the meantime, I see a 67-year-old white male with pain at base of penis for the last 2-3 days. It has him rolling on the ground in pain. He has a very tender prostate gland on rectal exam, and has a pretty obvious case of prostatitis.

Prostatitis is typically a bacterial infection. In young men it's usually caused by chlamydia (a sexually transmitted disease). In older folks it's usually due to a gut contaminant E. coli. It produces acute and chronic pain at the base of the penis. It responds to antibiotics, but frequently recurs.

I give this guy a shot of Demerol (a big gun narcotic), and start him on Levaquin (an antibiotic) and Vicodin (a mild narcotic). He already has an appointment with his urologist, and this should get him through the weekend.

Our 14-year-old makes it back from Radiology and his films are fine. I talk him into letting me repair his face, then I spend a half hour or so putting it back together. His bill from this would likely make a serious down payment on another 4-wheeler. It would definitely buy a few dozen of the helmets that might have prevented the injury.

Okay, then we have 25-year-old white female who's 8-10 weeks pregnant, and is cramping and spotting. She's here wanting an ultrasound.

I have a standard spiel I give these girls about how 10-15% of all pregnancies end in miscarriage in the first 3 months. Usually it's a genetic problem of some type. There's nothing that can be done one way or the other. The standard stuff...

The bottom line is that if the local obstetricians won't take care of their patients after hours, then the path of least resistance is to give them what they want. They want reassurance that the pregnancy is going okay, and an ultrasound is the best way I'm able to go about it.

Uuup, we have a positive Samsonite sign. It's a little old lady, in no distress, who's here with her bag in hand. It's an 87-year-old white female who tells me she was diagnosed with pneumonia earlier in the week, and was started on an antibiotic and a cough medicine. She has been getting weaker despite her current treatment. The goal, in order to meet her agenda, is to find an admission criteria so we can keep her. We'll see...

9:00 PM

In the meantime, all hell is breaking loose. The town is waking up, and they all need to be touched by a doctor.

First, I see a 2-month-old white male with a week of fussiness. It's a kid I passed off last week at shift change that turned out to have influenza A. The child has been colicky, and has been in to see his regular doctor almost daily, including this morning. They are just convinced that something is seriously wrong with their little one. My job becomes one of torturing the kid with tests until I've done enough to convince the parents that their little bundle of joy is going to return to being a bundle of joy rather than a demon child from hell. Now, I really need to be doing testing on the parents. They're hardly more than kids themselves, and are obviously clueless.

It turns out we've struck it rich on our little grandma with the positive bag sign. She is pretty hypoxic (her oxygen level is low), and meets criteria for needing supplemental oxygen. This in itself provides a reason for admission. Her heart doesn't seem to like the low oxygen either, and she's got some new changes on her EKG as well. We're swamped, so I call her doctor early and get her admitted.

Second is a 26-year-old white female who's had a fever for the last several days. She was seen yesterday, had a negative influenza screen, and told she has a virus. She continues to have a fever. As a child she had a febrile seizure, and she's sure she is going to have one now. She's got a whopping 2-degree fever! (Yawn)

Well, febrile seizures are common with temperatures over 104, IN CHILDREN UNDER 2 YEARS OF AGE. In fact, they can occur in something like 5% of kids with very high temps. They really don't mean anything, and they don't occur in adults. I'm sure it has something to do with the development stage of a youthful brain, and the like.

Well, it takes me quite a while to convince this person that she's going to be fine. The fever will run its course, and she'll get better. She still seems kind of skeptical when she leaves, but there's not much I can do about that.

Well, let's go back to our 2-month-old for a while. Everything I do is normal. A set of belly films shows a lot of gas, which is likely where the colicky pain is coming from. I discuss the case at some length with the regular doctor, who'd seen the kid this morning. He agrees with me that the child is fine, and that it's the parents that need work. We finally settle on changing to a new hypoallergenic formula, in case there is a component of formula intolerance. I spend ages trying to reassure the parents, and I send them on their way. Whew…

Third is the more mundane. It's a 17-year-old white female who twisted her ankle playing basketball. Her films are normal, and she is sent with routine sprain instructions.

Fourth we get a 95-year-old white female in by squad. She'd been having increasing back pain for the last week, and it's a crisis now. It's admirable that she has been able to live independently for so long, but her days outside of a nursing home are numbered. I do quite a work-up, and don't find much except a boatload of arthritis. We try and get her up, but it's not going to fly. In the end, we wind up admitting her over night. She'll go to a nursing home tomorrow.

Fifth is a 12-month-old white male with a fever and a cough. The kid has just finished two courses of antibiotics for ear infection. Once again I'm dealing with parents who are convinced there is something seriously wrong with their kid, and in reality the kid just has a cold.

I'm faced with torturing and irradiating him to prove he's fine. I find nothing. They're sure the child needs to be in the hospital, but I'm not finding anything close to a criterion. In the end, I provide some reassurance that I'm not sure is effective, and recommend they check in with their regular doctor the first of the week.

Sixth is a 14-year-old white female who also twisted her ankle playing basketball. She wasn't as lucky, and broke it in two places. The orthopedic surgeon splints her, but will take her to surgery in the morning.

Seventh is a 15-year-old white female with a distant history of seizure. She's being weaned off her seizure medicines, and has had a couple of seizures at this lower dose. Sounds like she needs more meds! I contact her neurologist and bump her meds back up. Her parents could have done this just as easily from home, but whatever.

Eighth is a 14-year-old with wrist and forearm pain after wrestling this morning. His films are fine. He gets sprain instructions, and is sent on his way.

Ninth is a 19-year-old white male with a headache for 20 minutes. He is dramatic to beat the band, and acts like he's dying. He does have a bit of an ear infection. He's telling me that this is the worst headache of his life, so I'm obligated to scan his head. I'm sure it's going to be normal. I give him some routine headache medicine in the meantime. He's had some vomiting, so I give him Nubain (a non-narcotic pain medicine) and Phenergan (an antiemetic).

Tenth is a 50-year-old white male who comes in by squad with knee pain for a day. He twisted it this morning and wants to be admitted. This is just nuts. His exam is fine, as is a set of films. He's just sprained it. I also give him some Nubain (a non-narcotic pain medicine) and Phenergan (an anti-nausea medicine). I get him set up with a knee immobilizer and something for discomfort. He's already on an anti-inflammatory. He can check in with his orthopedic surgeon first of the week.

With all this going, midnight has rolled right up. My relief is here. I check out what I've got left and head upstairs to find a hospital bed.

There are no patients on the pediatrics floor, so I have the whole floor to myself.

12:00 AM

Zzzz...

Shift 11

"Macho medicine!"

Sunday—18 Hours

6:00 AM

Well, the morning came way too soon. I forgot my pager at home yesterday, and that's what I use as my alarm clock. I had to figure out how to use my PDA as an alarm. This was a challenge of its own after slaving away for 18 odd hours.

And we start out pretty much in high gear. The department is full, but most are just being discharged. It sounds like it was pretty miserable night.

We begin with a 19-year-old white female with several hours of abdominal pain. It's crampy, and seems to come and go. It all seems to be left sided. Her exam in pretty unremarkable, but she acts like she's dying. I give her a whiff of Demerol, and start our routine abdominal pain work-up. We'll see what we find.

Next is a 48-year-old white female who has had sinus drainage and a cough for several days. Since last evening she's also had some bladder pressure, and is concerned that she may have a bladder infection. A urinalysis is cooking.

Meanwhile there's an 8-year-old white female who ran into a pole and split open the area just below her eyebrow. It's amenable to Dermabond (skin glue), but she spazzes out just the same. I can't imagine what it would have taken to put stitches in this kid.

We also have 25-year-old white male with a "migraine" headache. This is yet another of our frequent flyers. He used to be big on demanding Demerol, but now takes what we give him. I give him our usual cocktail, and he's sent on his way.

Our 48-year-old with the bladder pressure has a normal urinalysis. She's still convinced she has a bladder infection despite the lack of findings. He symptoms are probably related to her coughing. I cover her with an antibiotic, as she's expecting it. I give her some symptomatic medicines as well.

Our 19-year-old with the belly pain is now feeling no pain and is sleeping. Everything is coming back normal. She has been on multiple medicines for a presumed sinus infection, many of which can have GI side effects. In the end it looks like that's all that's going on. Well, that and being a reactive, dramatic 19-year-old.

We then start seeing our ice casualties. I guess folks are starting to wake up and fall down. It's a 35-year-old white female who fell on the ice and twisted her ankle. She's weight bearing without difficulty and has a normal exam. Whatever happened to the days when people realized they've twisted their ankle, and waited more than 30 minutes before racing in to get a x-ray. Of course her films are normal, and I treat her like a sprain.

Then there's a 45-year-old white female who scratched her eye yesterday. Now its red, mattery, and painful. From the look of it, it's obviously infected. When I put in some fluorescein dye, there is a huge corneal abrasion that lights up under UV light. I put her on some Tobrex drops (an antibiotic) and some Vicprofen (a mild narcotic). She should be fine in a day or so.

There's a 14-year-old white female with cold symptoms for a week and ear pain for a day. She does have an ear infection. I put her on some Amoxicillin (an antibiotic), and send her on her way.

Boy, we are off to the races.

First, I see a 9-month-old white male with a runny nose and a cough for a day. The kid looks fine except for a snotty nose. It's definitely not an emergency. The kid's got a cold. I give the mom some antihistamine/decongestant drops for him, so it seems like I'm doing something, and send them along.

Second is a 4-year-old white female with a fever and sore throat since this morning. Her strep test is negative. This is another non-emergency that could have waited till tomorrow when the clinics opened. It's treated symptomatically.

Third is a 2-year-old white male with a recurrent cough for 2 months. The cough is worse for the last two days. The kid looks fine, but the mother is completely decompensating. She demands a chest x-ray. Normal! The kid goes to day care, and is probably picking up a range of viral bugs along the way. They want aggressive treatment, so I put the kid on some Pediapred (a steroid) to appease the parents.

It's amazing how much we have to torture and irradiate children simply to convince parents that their child is fine. There just seems to be so many folks who apparently want their child to be severely ill. I don't understand it. Common sense seems to be absent. There also seems to be an erroneous impression that medical science has a "cure" for everything, and if they don't leave with that cure, then they are somehow getting substandard care. Well, the reality is that a lot of childhood illness is viral, and we don't have antiviral meds to cover them all. For the most part though, these bugs are self-limited and only need supportive care.

Fourth is a 77-year-old white female who put her hand in a meat slicer. She nipped off a pretty good chunk of her finger, but it really doesn't leave much to sew. It gets a dressing, and will heal in 3-4 weeks.

Fifth is a 4-year-old white male who was being carried by his father when dad slipped on the ice. They went down together, and the kid wound up with quite a bruise on his penis. He's otherwise fine. This will heal in a week or two. The kids a little sore, but otherwise fine.

Sixth is the 28-year-old white male who's the father that fell with his kid. He racked out his knee in the fall. I get some films, but they're normal. He's just bruised it. Some crutches, an ace wrap, and an anti-inflammatory is all that he really needs. He'll live.

12:00 PM

Not really much opportunity to get lunch, as folks keep pouring on in.

Seventh is a 7-year-old white female with cough and congestion for a day. The kid has a cold. I check an influenza and strep screen just so it looks like I'm doing something, but there is absolutely no reason for her to be here.

Eighth is a 25-year-old white female with wrist pain for a day. She has no history of trauma, and hasn't really bothered to take anything for it. The exam is normal except for some minimal tenderness over some of the tendons. If she'd taken some Motrin or Aleve she wouldn't need to have come in here.

Ninth is a 19-month-old female whose mother slipped on the ice. The child was caught, but still managed to bop the back of her head. She was stunned for a minute or so, but didn't go completely out. She's been fine since. The parents are not going to be satisfied unless a head scan is done. It really isn't needed, and the child certainly doesn't need all the radiation she'll get from a CT, but it'll save same complaints, law suits etc. In the end, of course, it's normal.

Tenth is a 30-year-old white female with intermittent flank pain for a month. It's worse today. She's never had it evaluated anytime in the last month. Shortly after she arrives, her pain in gone. The nurse had gotten a urinalysis, and she does have quite a bit of blood. She's likely had some small kidney stones. We'll have her push fluids, strain her urine for stones, and follow-up with her doctor on Monday.

Eleventh is a 12-year-old white male with a sore throat and cough for a day. We seem to be having a trend here. I check a strep and influenza screen and they're negative. It's another boy with a cold.

Twelfth is a 19-year-old white male with chest wall pain for a week. He lifts heavy boxes at work. The area is tender. He's just overdone it. Of course he's not taken anything for this, nor has he contacted his regular doctor. In the end, the real agenda is a work release. Fine! Whatever he wants.

Thirteenth is a 30-year-old white male with tooth pain. He cracked a tooth a month ago, and didn't bother having it taken care of. It's a crisis now. It looks infected, so he needs an antibiotic. It's not painful enough that he will allow me to inject it with Novocaine. That would make it immediately pain free. He leaves with a few pain pills and an antibiotic.

It's a frequent ploy of drug seekers to come in complaining of tooth pain. Nine times out of ten they are snaggle tooth folks anyway, so they could be having tooth pain. I just hope a day comes where we have an objective way to assess pain.

I sometimes joke about my own special pain scale. Usually, pain is rated by a patient on a scale of 1 to 10. 10 is the worst pain of their life. I comment that I would come in with pruning sheers. I take off a finger at a time. The little finger is a one, and you move across to a maximum of ten. For those folks who say they are having pain in excess of the maximum 10, I'll start work on their toes. Somehow I don't think I'll have many folks with pain greater than a 1.

Fourteenth is a 44-year-old white female with pain from an abdominal incision. She had had an ovary removed, and is having pain at one edge of the incision. I do some basic lab. A worrisome thing could be an abscess or incarcerated loop of bowel. The patient is way too dramatic to tell how much pain she's really having. I send her off to CT to get a good look through the area.

Fifteenth is a 29-year-old white female who punctured her hand on a piece of glass while pushing down the garbage at home. This happened last night, and she's concerned that it's becoming infected. I explore the wound for glass, and don't find any. It really doesn't look infected, but I put her on an antibiotic because it's what she expects.

Sixteenth is an 11-year-old white female with fever, cough, and congestion for a day. It's the same stuff, different time. She does test positive for influenza, so I put her on Flumadine (an antiviral influenza medicine).

Antiviral treatment for influenza is vastly overrated. It costs a lot, has a very high incidence of GI side effects, and only reduces the course of the disease by a day or so. This is hardly a good tradeoff. It seems to me that a influenza vaccination is a better choice.

Seventeenth is a 71-year-old white female with back pain. This has been going on for months, and she's under treatment for it already. "It's not any better!" She's here because she wants it x-rayed. Fine! That's the path of least resistance. Of course it's normal for age. There's a lot of arthritis. She is scheduled to see her doctor in the morning, so doesn't want anything more for it. She just wanted the x-ray, and is then ready to go.

Back to our 44-year-old with the incisional pain. Her lab and her scan are normal. She's scheduled to see her regular doctor in the morning. It's likely a nerve pain from where the nerve endings were cut in the surgery. I give her some pain pills, and she can follow-up in the morning.

Eighteenth is a 26-year-old white female with abdominal pain. It began about 24 hours before with mid-abdominal pain and anorexia (doesn't feel like eating). Overnight it has migrated to the right lower quadrant. On exam, she has focal right lower abdominal tenderness. This is appendicitis until proven otherwise. She does have a low-grade fever. Her white count is elevated. Her other lab is normal. I call her regular doctor, and he concurs that it's an appy, as does the surgeon.

Many times the presentation of appendicitis is much less straightforward. In those cases I often do a pelvic CT scan. This can be up to 95% sensitive for appendicitis. It gets even more complicated when the patient is pregnant. You really can't do CT, so you have to either do the next best thing, ultrasound, or take her to the operating room.

Nineteenth is a 58-year-old white female, a 3 pack a day smoker, who's had a productive cough for three weeks. It's no worse today. It's forced her to cut back to a pack a day. She hasn't contacted her regular doctor at any time in the last three weeks, and she wants an antibiotic. I do a chest x-ray for good measure, and it just looks like a person who smokes three packs a day. I give her what she wants and send her along.

Twentieth is a 17-year-old white female with 1 week of sore throat and cough. We do an influenza screen and strep screen. The mother demands that we do a mono test as well. This is McMedicine, of course, so we do what she asks for. Everything's negative. She's got a virus, just not one we can test for. She needs to wait it out. She'll live.

Twenty-first is an 80-year-old white male with shortness of breath. This is a dialysis patient with a problem list as long as your arm. It could be anything, but he's likely in worsening heart failure. These folks have their fluid managed strictly by the dialysis. They usually have their dialysis three times a week, typically Monday, Wednesday, and Friday. This means that they go two days on the weekend without dialysis. This is also the time when they are more likely to eat and drink more than they should. They become fluid overloaded, and wind up in heart failure. We typically see these folks Sunday night, and this guy is right on schedule.

The only real fix for these patients is early dialysis. Their kidneys don't work, so diuretics (water pills) are not an effective solution. The severity of the fluid overload determines whether a person needs immediate dialysis, or whether it can wait a day or so. In this fellow, we'll see.

Twenty-second is a 16-year-old white male who twisted his ankle playing basketball. His films are fine, he's out of here.

6:00 PM

Surprisingly, there's a slight lull around the evening meal. There's some big football game that has just started, so that's probably what's going on. Things can't be a crisis during the game, it's always before or after.

Our 80-year-old with the shortness of breath is in some failure. Everything else is as normal as a dialysis patient can be. His oxygen saturations are fine. He should be able to go home and have his regular dialysis in the morning.

Sheee's back! The 26-year-old that I saw earlier with the probable kidney stone is back with increasing pain. It looks like it's time to do more. I have an IV started, and give fluids and Toradol (an anti-inflammatory). Once we get kidney function lab back, she heads off to Radiology for an IVP (a dye study looking for kidney stones).

Meanwhile, I see a 39-year-old white female who sliced her finger on a broken dish while doing dishes. She's completely avulsed a strip of tissue at the tip of the finger. There's really nothing left to sew. It just needs a Band-Aid.

There's a 23-year-old white male with a sore spot on his ear for three days. He tells me, "I was worried that it would make me go deaf." This is a real head scratcher to me. How a sore area that's not much bigger than the head of a pin could do that, I wouldn't know. Some folks think the weirdest things. When I look at it, I really don't see much of anything. It's a tender spot on his ear. He can keep an eye on it. I try and reassure him that his hearing is safe.

The next patient has a common complaint, especially on a weekend. It's a 40-year-old white female asthmatic who tells me she ran out of her medicines. These folks usually come in after the pharmacies are closed, knowing that we are obligated to supply them. It's frequently folks that can't or don't want to buy their medicines. It torques my jaws when these folks have a pack of cigarettes in their pockets. Well, I give her the meds and send her on her way. It's an awfully expensive way to get medicine refills.

Then we're back to the theme of the day. It's a 9-month-old white female with a fever and cough. She has a negative strep and influenza screen. She's got a cold. Deal with it.

This is followed immediately by a 4-year-old white male with, guess what? A fever and cough. It's the same song, different verse.

I see an 80-year-old non-compliant diabetic who is dizzy and confused. Well, she's always confused, and she's frequently dizzy. Her average blood sugar on her home glucose meter is just under 300 (normal is

65-120). I do a range of stuff, and all I find is that she is slightly dehydrated. She needs to drink more, be more compliant with her meds, and the like.

My last patient of the day is a 3-year-old white female who managed go get a plastic clip stuck on her tooth. As you might imagine, she is spazzing out to beat the band. In this job you have to be innovative to deal with these things. I finally manage to get two clamps on it, and twist it off. Whew…

My replacement is here, and I am gone…

12:00 AM

Shift 12

"Hot lights and cold steel..."

Tuesday—18 Hours

6:00 AM

I arrive to an empty ER. I spent the night in town as there was a winter storm warning, and I didn't want to try driving 60 miles through blizzard conditions at 3:00 a.m. It was sleeting all day yesterday, and there is a nice half-inch of ice under the snow.

Of course, consistent with my black cloud, there's a pedi call almost immediately. The answering service of a local pediatrics group is sending in a kid with hives. It's not more than 30 seconds later when the family arrives. It's a 2-year-old white male. He does have some hives and some minimal angioedema (facial soft tissue swelling). The family is acting like the child's dying. The kid's in more distress from all the commotion being made than about the hives and whatnot. I give him some Benadryl (an antihistamine) and some Pediapred (a steroid), and we watch him for a while.

Next is an 86-year-old white female. She slipped and fell at home, hurting her hip and ankle. She's in by squad. We film everything that hurts, and she did manage to break her ankle.

This is followed immediately by a 68-year-old white female who has a hip prosthesis that may have spontaneously dislocated. She's also in by squad. I give her some IV Demerol to get her comfortable enough to get her filmed.

Our 86-year-old was recently started on a combination diabetes medicine. She tells us she has intermittent episodes of shakiness. Her blood sugar this morning was 45, which is enough to make a person shaky. I chat with her regular doctor and the orthopedic surgeon. We decrease her blood sugar medicine, and put a walking boot on her foot.

An 18-year-old white male follows this. He's depressed, and wants to die. It sounds like there have been a lot of social stresses, problems with parents, problems at school, and the like. Sometimes you just want to tell these kids to suck it up and get with the program. This is a middle-class kid. How bad can life be? We get the police involved to get a hold on him; this gives us the ability to hold him against his will if he should try and bolt. We then start trying to coordinate a psychiatric facility to accept him for evaluation.

I also see a 39-year-old white female with our first "migraine" headache of the day. She tells me she would have gone to see her regular doctor, but the weather is too bad. Fine! It's pretty nasty out there, so I'll give her the benefit of the doubt.

There's also an 81-year-old white female with right flank pain for the last 4-5 days. It's much better today, so she came in the ER. I'm not quite sure what the logic is here. She does have a history of multiple abdominal surgeries, so the list of possibilities is significant. I start my routine abdominal evaluation, and we've see...

It sounds like a squad's inbound from a local assisted living facility with someone with breathing problems...

And the answer is...It's a 91-year-old white female who's pretty much demented and deaf as a stump. She's been refusing her medicines for some time, smoking like a chimney, and now she's short of breath. It's like, what chronic disease doesn't she have? She has chronic heart disease, lung disease, recurrent gastrointestinal bleed, and the list goes on. The family is fixated on her being anemic. They tell me that the last time she was like this she needed a transfusion. Okay, well maybe. It's best to not get tunnel vision about this. Her lungs sound like crap, likely from all the smoking, so I get her a breathing treatment. Her oxygen level is fine. I start a cardiac work-up just for good measure, and we'll see what we find.

Meanwhile I see the next train wreck. It's a 65-year-old white male with advanced lung cancer. He's been getting chemotherapy, and has been puking his guts out since then. He's also feeling more short of breath this morning, and just in general is feeling progressively weaker. Add to this that the family pulls me off to the side to let me know he's just too much to handle at home. Hmmm, real supportive family we've got here. These folks don't realize that he's not going to be cured with the chemo, and his life expectancy is such that he shouldn't be making any long-term plans. This guys lungs sound like crap, and my initial impression is that he's probably got a post obstructive pneumonia; this is a pneumonia that can occur when the cancer blocks off a large airways in the lung, and the obstructed area becomes infected. He does have a bit of a fever as well. I get him a breathing treatment, and start the work-up…

12:00 PM

I brought some cans of soup from home, which is a good thing. Trying to maintain a low fat diet on hospital cafeteria food is almost impossible. You would think that organizations that are tasked with looking after folk's health would set better examples. The same could also be said of hospital personnel with other bad habits, like smoking and the like. I really don't understand it.

Well we start to get information back on our 91-year-old. It looks like she's in heart failure. She's got quite a bit a fluid built up in her lungs. It seems she quit taking her diuretic (water pill) early in the scheme of things, because it made her pee too much. I'm sure part of it is also bronchitis from her smoking. She's anemic, but this has been stable and is not at a level requiring transfusion. I give her some Lasix (a diuretic) in her IV and chat with her regular doctor. All of her problems are really ones of noncompliance. We can't force her to take her meds. We restart her on all the appropriate stuff and send her back home. She may take it for a while, and is then likely to be right back here. Even if she was in a more structured environment, like a nursing home, you can't force a person to do something they don't want to do. In a 91-year-old, you could argue that you don't have the right to even try.

I see a 72-year-old white female with palpitations. She has herself worked up into a frenzy. I do an EKG, and it's completely normal. I do a range of cardiac lab that is normal as well. She has one of her spells while in the ER, while on the monitor. Her rhythm is completely normal, but she has a muscle in her left chest that's twitching. Her palpitations are really just a muscle twitch and not cardiac at all. I do a holter monitor just for good measure (an ambulatory heart monitor that is worn for 24 hours), and send her on her way.

Back to our 65-year-old lung cancer patient. I've given him some fluids and some Zofran (an anti-nausea medicine that's effective for chemotherapy associated vomiting). His chest x-ray looks okay except for the huge mass of cancer. He's got a sodium level that's subterranean. This is a common problem with lung malignancies via an interaction with the kidneys known as SIADH (syndrome of inappropriate antidiuretic hormone). I chat with his regular doctor. He'll be admitted for tune-up, and then sent off to the nursing home. It's too bad that death can't be a bit tidier.

It seems to be the day for palpitations, and my next patient is a case in point. It's a 25-year-old white female with, you guessed it, palpitations. I do an EKG, and surprisingly enough she's in atrial fibrillation (an arrhythmia). This is pretty unusual in someone so young, and is frequently associated with cocaine and methamphetamine abuse in this age range. Regardless, it has the same risks to the patient. The biggest long-term risk is a 5% annual stroke risk. This almost guarantees an early stroke in someone this young unless they are either converted back to a normal rhythm or put on some form of stroke prevention. She is a regular of doctor NONE, so I call the on-call doctor early and get her admitted.

My next case I find pathetic. It's a 38-year-old white female who slipped on the ice in front of a local business and bumped her arm. It's fine, just bruised. Her comment to me is that she's glad that she fell on the business property because now she can sue them.

Whatever happened to the days when folks took responsibility for their actions, and recognized that life has some inherent risks. It seems that so many people want to play the litigation lottery. They go looking for a reason to sue people so they can get the easy money. It's unfortunate that there are so many lawyers out there that facilitate this behavior. Ah well, so much for my soapbox.

Back into the fray with a "real" emergency. It's a 45-year-old white female with her usual "migraine" headache. It is just too inconvenient for her to see her regular doctor. She doesn't want to have to drive in the weather, so she's come to see us. She gets the usual.

The way I see it we should only ever see a person once for a true migraine headache, and that's the first headache. From that point on, they should be working through their regular doctor. I'm sorry but migraine headaches are really NOT emergencies. Although, I could say the same about 95% of everything that shows up in the ER these days.

I get a little break in the action, and get caught up on the paperwork. Then it's time for fruits, nuts, and fender benders. My next patient hits all these categories. It's a 45-year-old white female who lost control of her vehicle on the ice. She's bipolar, manic to beat the band, and obviously not well medicated. She tells me that everything hurts, so I'm faced with irradiating her till she glows in the dark, x-raying all her aches and pains. It's hard to get a word in edgewise with this lady.

Bipolar disorder is a common psychiatric problem. It's characterized by swings from mania to depression. During mania, a patient may become grandiose, and impulsive. They might go into a store and buy everything that takes their fancy, regardless of their ability to pay. During their depressive phase, they may become suicidal. These mood swings can be managed with medications, but the problem with a lot of psychiatric patients is that they frequently don't think there's anything wrong with them, and so they don't take their medicines.

I move from this to the more sublime. It's an 8-month-old white female with a fever for less than an hour. The mom wants a script for Tylenol. It's our Medicaid tax dollars at work. Well, the kid does have an ear infection, so I put her on an antibiotic as well.

It never ceases to amaze me the sheer numbers of able-bodied adults on Welfare, Medicaid, and the like. We're in the best economic times in the history of the nation, when businesses can't find enough people to work for them, and there's a large group of people who apparently don't want to work.

Well, back to it. My next challenge is a 25-year-old mentally retarded white male who had just been discharged from the hospital less than an hour before. He's apparently having increased abdominal pain. He was in with severe constipation that took days to get taken care of. Stepping into the room was like stepping into a hornet's nest naked. The family did everything short of handing me my head on a platter. They are very upset that the patient was released before he was all-better, and are taking it out on me. I've not even seen this patient before. I order a shotgun of stuff to try and sort out what may be going on. Then the family is upset that I'm going to have blood drawn from this guy. This is definitely a no win situation. I finally convince these folks to let me do my job, and assure them that I'll be in constant contact with their regular doctor (who dumped this into my lap).

Okay, back to our 45-year-old crazy person. She's finally back from Radiology. If you use your imagination you can see her lightly glowing from all the irradiation. About 50 films were done, and surprise, they're normal. Then it's a matter of hustling her out the door, finally…

Our next casualty is a 16-year-old who got head butted by his friend while wrestling. His nose seems a bit off centered. Once we get the films, it does look fractured. However, this is really not an emergency. It needs two or three days for the swelling to go down, then the ENT folks can do something with it, if necessary.

I see an 8-year-old white female who got in the way of her brother's show shovel. She's got a left eyebrow laceration. It's amenable to Dermabond (skin glue), and she's on her way.

There's a 70-year-old white female who's had a finger infection for 4 months, and has been under treatment with antibiotics for that whole time. She was supposed to go to an appointment with her orthopedic doctor to follow-up on this, but didn't want to make the trip because of the ice and snow on the road. It's really no worse, but she shows up in my ER rather than to her doctor appointment. She has been going some distance to see this other doctor, but she wants stay more local in her future dealings. Why is this an emergency? Who knows? I have no records on her, so I have to begin an evaluation from the beginning. Of course, she has no idea what medicines or antibiotics she's on, and she's on a boatload. I order a film and some lab. Given the duration of her infection, she probably has involvement of the underlying bone.

While I'm waiting, I see a 29-year-old white female who apparently hurt her back at work this morning. I figure out pretty quickly that the real agenda is that she wants a few days off from work. Such an expensive way to go about it, but fine.

I also see a 57-year-old white female with two hours of pain and burning with urination. Her urinalysis is strongly positive, so I put her on an appropriate antibiotic (Bactrim) for a week. In younger women you can usually get away with three days, but I've seen too many treatment failures when older folks are treated with such a short course.

Then I'm back to pediatrics with a 4-year-old white female with a red bump on her eyelid. It's a hordeolum, or stye. It's just a local infection of a gland in the eyelid. Hot-packs are all it really takes, but the parents want her on an antibiotic, so I put her on some Zithromax (an antibiotic).

Our final case before dinner is a 9-year-old white female with our familiar theme of fever, sore throat, and cough. Her strep and influenza screens are negative, as is her exam. She's yet another with "the bug." It needs to be treated symptomatically.

6:00 PM

Boring, boring food.

And we're back into it with a 26-year-old white female who slipped on the ice and twisted her ankle. It's yet another normal x-ray.

Then there's a 37-year-old white female asthmatic with increasing shortness of breath. She's feeling much better after a shot of Solu-Medrol (a steroid) and multiple breathing treatments. Her chest x-ray is normal. She's already on Biaxin (an antibiotic adequate for pneumonia). I change her inhaler to Combivent (a two-medicine inhaler, Ventolin and Atrovent), put her on an extended course of prednisone (a steroid), and send her on her way.

Then we have another ice casualty. It's a 48-year-old white male who fell in his drive and scraped his scalp on his car. He needs three skin staples to put him back together.

The next patient takes the cake for our cavalcade of fruits and nut. It's a 25-year-old white male who comes in by squad after a supposed insect bite. This person is just downright bizarre. The area he points to has no sign of having been bitten, nor is there any local or systemic sign of an allergic reaction. I offer a shot of medicine to reverse allergic reactions, but he refuses. I give him some Benadryl (an antihistamine) and some Prednisone (a steroid), and he immediately acts like he's having some type of reaction to the medicine after he swallows them. Again, there is no objective evidence to support this. Then he proceeds to go into my "globally positive review of systems." Literally everything that could hurt does hurt, every symptom he could have he does have. This guy is a nut with a capital "N." Now what the secondary gain is, I don't know. I've rapidly satisfied myself that he has no threatening problem, and have my nurse shoe him out the door. I wonder if this guy is going to be another frequent flyer.

Let's get back to the worried well. Next is a 33-year-old white male who twisted his knee. He's tender, but his films are fine. He acts like his leg was ripped off. It's a sprain, show some backbone! This is a real big, athletic, macho dude, and he's acting like a baby. I treat him for his sprain and send him on his way.

We're then back to fruits and nuts. It's a 22-year-old white male who got in a verbal fight with a family member, and they winged a dish at him. It struck him in the ankle, and he's barely even got a visible bruise there. He comes in by squad, and gets the police involved. He demands that the other party be arrested. I do a film and it's normal. This is pathetic! He's now managed to generate a $1000+ bruise with all the resources he's sequestered with his little temper tantrum.

Well, time for a new theme. It's a 40-year-old white female with diarrhea for a day, and cramping for twenty minutes. The cramping is gone by the time I see her. She's another one who acts like she's dying. I do routine abdominal stuff, and it's normal. She's got the stomach bug. She'll live. The pain was likely gas.

Back to pediatrics and a 3-year-old white female with ear pain. She's got an ear infection, and I start her on some Amoxicillin (an antibiotic).

There's a 20-month-old white female who had vomited 4 or 5 times in rapid succession. With the last emesis there may have been some trace blood. The kid's happy, playful, and racing around the room. She likely had some esophageal irritation. She is sent with routine vomiting instructions.

I also see a 28-year-old white female with diarrhea all day, and twenty minutes of right sided cramping. This is yet one more person who acts like they're going to die. Everything is normal, except her belly films show she's packed with poop. Her pain is cured after she has a large spontaneous BM in the ER. Yawn, what an emergency.

Then it's a 3-year-old hispanic male with a rash since this morning. He's got a few hives, and so I put him on some Benadryl (an antihistamine). Before they go, the family asks if they can have some free vitamins. Yeah, right!

I also see a 14-year-old white male with asthma. He was diagnosed with influenza yesterday, and is complaining of chest pain with breathing and shortness of breath. Every measure of asthma severity is normal. Chest pain and cough are expected symptoms with influenza.

I give him Tessilon (a cough medicine) for cough, and some Darvocet (a mild narcotic) for his pain.

My last patient of the day has to be yet another nut. It's a 33-year-old white male with dry mouth, tingling face and arms, racing heart, and the like. He's another who's sure he's going to die. An EKG is completely normal. This guy is a recovering methamphetamine addict, and he's got about a million stresses in his life. He's hyperventilating, and having an anxiety attack. It turns out he's had problems with anxiety attacks before. He's pretty much cured with my talking to him, and down right mellow after a Xanax (a tranquilizer). I give him a few Xanax, and send him on his way. He can follow-up with his regular doctor if he needs something more.

Well, the witching hour has arrive, and with it my relief. I'm out of here and up to a hospital bed for my meager five hours or so of sleep.

12:00 AM

Zzzz...

Shift 13

"Death and destruction..."

Wednesday—18 Hours

6:00 AM

I sleep like the dead. That's one of the strange things about a career in medicine. You learn how to sleep pretty much anywhere, any time. I can get pretty comfortable in a hospital bed. Granted, I'd rather be at home, but I can make due with most anything.

I thought I was saved. A woman having chest pain walks in with one of the local doctors. It looks like he's going to take care of her, but it turns out he's headed off to a meeting.

It's a 70-year-old white female with one hour of left sided chest pain. For the last several months she's been having exertional chest pain. This is the first time she's had pain without exertion. This lady has absolutely no past medical history. Her EKG shows subtle change in the area associated with the inferior part of the heart. She is given an aspirin, put on oxygen, and given nitroglycerine. With these maneuvers, she's pain free. I give other protective meds for good measure. This is cardiac pain until proven otherwise. Routine cardiac stuff is ordered. Then we mark time waiting for the regular doctor to finish his meeting. Ah well, I'd rather be doing this than all of the cough and runny nose stuff.

Once my chest pain is stabilized, I nip off to see an 18-year-old white male who put his arm through a plate glass window. He came real close to doing himself some real damage, but in the end it is just a flesh wound. I wind up closing it with two layers of sutures, but it'll be fine.

My next victim is a 32-year-old white male with upper abdominal pain. He has a history of bad gastroesophageal reflux (GERD), and has had a surgery to try and fix this (a Nissen fundoplication).

A Nissen uses the upper part of the stomach and wraps it around the esophagus to make a new lower esophageal valve. One of the problems with this is that it frequently makes it impossible to vomit.

Well this guy has had a stomach bug for the last several days, has been nauseated, and has been trying to vomit. This has produced severe upper abdominal pain due to esophageal irritation. We do routine abdominal and cardiac things that ensure nothing else is going on, and they're all-normal. His pain responds to Zantac (an acid blocker). I put him on high dose Prilosec (a stronger acid blocker) with instructions to follow-up as necessary.

Meanwhile we have a work-place injury. It's a 45-year-old white male that mashed his little toe at work. His film is normal, and he's only got a superficial abrasion visible. This is treated symptomatically and he's sent on his way.

Wouldn't you know it though, the squad is inbound with a hip pain. There was apparently a fall at one of the nursing homes.

It's no sooner that they encode that they arrive. It's a 75-year-old white female who had taken a ground level fall in the home. She's having a lot of hip pain, and is writhing on the cart. Her affected leg does appear somewhat shorter, and it is rotated. I'm betting she has a fractured hip. I have the nurse give her some Demerol (a strong narcotic), and she's whisked down to Radiology.

Before they go, the squad guys say that there's another squad coming in with a difficulty breathing. Oh joy.

And the answer is…It's a 75-year-old white female who's had a bad stomach bug with diarrhea. When they load her she promptly vomits and then aspirates. Her oxygen level drops to a point where she needs supplemental oxygen. She has a 102 fever, and is pretty obtunded (difficult to arouse). We get her on some oxygen, and get her a breathing treatment. We'll see what else we find.

Next is an 80-year-old white male who has had some rectal pain and noticed some blood on his sheets. This guy has thumb sized hemorrhoids, but is otherwise normal. This is not something I'm going to fix, and neither is it a threat. I give him some Anusol HC (a hemorrhoid cream). He can see one of the surgeons if he wants them removed.

Then there's a 21-year-old white male smoker. He's had chest pain and tenderness for 3 day. He rates his pain a 20 on a scale of 1 to 10. Right! I don't think so. This is another case where I want to use my finger and toe scale. He's sure that he's dying. His EKG is normal, as is his chest x-ray. I do a knee-jerk influenza screen as well, and it's negative. He's got tenderness over the cartilage in his left chest. This is costochondritis, a viral inflammation of the cartilage. It produces pain, and responds to anti-inflammatories. I put him on some Naproxen (an anti-inflammatory) and some Vicodin (a mild narcotic) and send him along.

Next in our drama series is a 28-year-old white female who lost control of her car on the ice, and slid into the ditch. She was restrained. There was no damage to the car, and it was driven out of the ditch. She tells me that she hurts pretty much everywhere. I can't very well film every bone in her body, she would glow white hot before I was done. We focus on the most painful areas, and send her on down to Radiology.

Then I move on to a 95-year-old white male who's been having bloody stools. On rectal exam there's lots of blood, and his blood count is about half of normal. Yup, I'd say he's doing some bleeding. A tube is put in his stomach to look for blood, and it's clear. He's given some IV fluids, IV Zantac (a stomach acid reducing medicine), and is typed and cross-matched for blood. The local doctor is contacted, and the patient is admitted.

12:00 PM

Lunch pretty much sucks except for the soup.

Then I'm back into the death and destruction. I see a 19-month-old white male who'd fallen flat on his face. He had some oral bleeding, and was brought in for evaluation. The bleeding is completely stopped when I see him. Except for some dried blood on his chin, and some superficial lip abrasions, he's completely normal.

Our car wreck victim finally gets back from Radiology. Of course everything is completely normal. She can treat all this symptomatically.

Then it's time for some real excitement. I get a 45-year-old white male, in by squad, who put a 16-penny nail into his upper arm with a nail gun. Oh joy. I sent him off for x-ray to see just where it's at. At first I feel kind of gutsy, and think I'll just pull it out. Then I start to think about just how long that nail is, and how many different structures are in the area.

Shortly thereafter, I see an 88-year-old white female who had slipped and fallen on the ice. It sounds, from the physical description of the foot right after the fall, that she had completely disarticulated her foot. Now it just kind of flops back and forth. I would venture a guess that it didn't do that before. The x-ray looks pretty disgusting. It's going to take an orthopedic surgeon to fix that.

Back to our guy who nailed himself, I call the orthopedic surgeon to take a look. My biggest fear is that I'd pull out that nail and start spraying the walls with his blood. Our surgeon throws caution to the wind, looks at the nail for a while, and just pulls it out. Wouldn't you know it, it starts bleeding to beat the band. It doesn't appear to be arterial, but it looks like he did clip a big pipe. This guy heads off to surgery, and our lady with the ankle is not far behind.

Then we're off to foolish accidents. It's a 25-year-old white female who managed to spill hot oil on her hand. She's got first and second degree burns to the back of the hand. No areas are circumferential. The wounds are cleaned and are dressed with Silvadene cream (a burn cream). She needs to have this looked at again in a day or two.

6:00 PM

Two squads are inbound with sledding injuries. We'll see...

And the answer is...There's a 14 and 15-year-old white male who lost control of their sled and hit a tree. The one in front, the 15-year-old, may have lost consciousness for a few seconds, and complains of neck and rib pain. The other complains of low back, and knee pain. They were both up at the scene, but subsequently brought in by squad on backboards and with cervical collars in place. Both their exams were unremarkable. I film their necks, and everything else that hurts. The one with the possible loss of consciousness gets a head CT scan as well. It's all-normal. It's just bumps and bruises. All in all, this makes for a very expensive sled outing. They are advised and sent home.

Hmmm...We seem to have another theme here. My next patient is a 7-year-old white male who lost control of his snowboard and struck his shoulder. And yes, it's broken. He's broken his clavicle! I put him in a clavicle strap (a belt arrangement that holds the shoulders back), and give him some Tylenol with codeine elixir for pain. He can follow-up with his regular doctor later in the week for a recheck.

I also see a 5-month-old white female who's had some breathing problems for the last 3 weeks. She's also had diarrhea for the last three days, and only wants to drink Pedialyte for the last day. The mom is spazzing out because she's sure the child is going to starve to death. She doesn't seem to realize that Pedialyte has quite a few calories. Also, a child is not going to starve to death in a day or two. This mom has been seeing a doctor once or twice a day. Let's look at the kid: she's happy, playful, and in no distress whatsoever. In the short time I see the child, she sucks down about 16 ounces of Pedialyte without a problem, and is happy as a clam. I do half hour or so of social work and reassurance, and finally (I think) convince the mom that the kid is going to be fine. Whew...

8:00 PM

Hmmm...We're having another lull. I'd be more than happy for this to go on till midnight. I only get six hours off, then I do one last 18 hour shift before my vacation. I am ready to get out of here now, I tell you. I just feel drained.

TV...

10:45 PM

Well, I guess it just couldn't last. A little 80-year-old white female was out on the town, and slipped on the ice. She's a mass of scrapes, and bruises, but nothing broken and no irreparable damages. We clean her up, update her tetanus, and send her on her way.

And then nothing. What a weird night!

Shift 14

"The end of my saga..."

Thursday—18 Hours

6:00 AM

I guess the weird night went on to be a weird early morning. There were only three patients overnight. This is unheard of on a weekday. A more normal number is 10 or 15. It was very cold and icy, so maybe people got smart.

Well, I start off with an ice injury. The first patient of the day, waiting just for me, is a 50-year-old white female who went down on the ice and snapped the bone in her lower leg in two places. She must have really come down hard. Both the tibia and the fibula are snapped in two and the ends are displaced. You usually see this in major trauma like car wrecks. Interesting, but a no brainer. I contact the orthopedic surgeon, and she's someone else's problem.

I've hardly finished with this gal, when we get our first chest pain of the day. It's pretty typical. They usually start rolling in first thing in the morning.

It's a 70-year-old white male with chest pain. He's a keeper.

Then it's just what I need, a 38-year-old white female drug seeking, chronic pain, fibromyalgia person with abdominal pain, back pain, throat pain, every pain. She's got the classic globally positive review of systems. Can you say nut? Looking at her record, she has had every test known to man. She's seen and alienated every physician in town, and seems to be working on adjacent towns. She's on a list of psychiatric and pain meds as long as your arm. The real question is, "what's her agenda?" She's already getting oral morphine for her various pain syndromes. I don't have anything stronger than this, nor would I give it to her if I did. She seems to want yet another work-up by yet another doctor to prove to her that she's okay. Fine! I can do it! I order a shotgun of tests to generally evaluate her back, abdomen, and whatnot. I know I won't find anything, but it could always save me a lawsuit.

Then it's time for the squads, and we get three in rapid succession.

First is a 30-year-old white male who was clipped by another car and went into the ditch in with his car. There was minimal damage to either car. He was up at the scene. When the police arrived, he decided he had neck pain. He is brought in on a backboard with a cervical collar in place. He makes a comment to the nurse that he hopes the other guy has lots of insurance. It seems like he wants to sue. From the sounds of it, it was an honest accident, and maybe even no-fault. Ah well, that's not my problem. I send him off to Radiology to film his normal neck.

Meanwhile, I see a 26-year-old white male who fell on the ice and rang his bell. Now he's got a 10 of 10 headache. I don't know, I'd still like to be able to use my finger pain scale. His exam is normal, but I become obligated to scan his head to prove there has been no bleed, so I send him along to Radiology as well.

While I'm waiting, I see a two-fer: a 38-year-old white female and her 39-year-old husband. They've both had cold symptoms for a few days. I do influenza screens for good measure, and they're negative. I send them with symptomatic meds. As they're being checked out, the real agenda surfaces. They both want work releases for the next few days. Fine, whatever!

Back to the others. Our 38-year-old has normal everything. I spend quite a long time providing reassurance that she's not going to die. I pretty much tell her that I don't have anything to offer her. She needs to manage her problems through her regular doctor. There's nothing life threatening going on, and that's all that I'm really concerned about.

Contrary to what a lot of folks think, and what television implies, the ER is very limited in what it can do. We are set up to find and temporize life-threatening things. Our mandate is not to necessarily figure out what is wrong, but just to figure out if it is a threat. If we choose to treat non-threatening, non-emergent, problems, it is more of a bonus to the patient than a requirement for us. It is the job of the primary care physician to figure out what is really going one, no matter how trivial, and to provide the appropriate treatment. Unlike us, they have all of medical science to draw from.

As for the other patients in progress…Our headache has a normal scan. I've given him some Toradol (an anti-inflammatory) and he's feeling better. I send him with a few pain pills and routine head instructions. Our neck pain has a normal set of neck films. He needs to take some Motrin or Aleve, and get a life. He's able bodied, but somehow managed to get on disability. I just hate these folks that game the system to get a handout. Ah well, nothing I do is going to change all that.

Well, let's see. Where are we?

The second squad brought up an 85-year-old white female with three days of fever and diarrhea. The family essentially says, "we'll stop by and pick her up in 4 or 5 days," and promptly leaves. Ah, I think not! The gal is pretty much bedridden at home, but about the only thing I see clinically is that she's a bit on the dry side. I start some intravenous fluids, and do some baseline lab. It's real questionable if I'm going to find an admission criteria, especially for 4 or 5 days. It's just not going to fly.

Folks seem to think that, because they have Medicaid, Medicare, or private insurance, they can obtain whatever medical services they want—on demand. It just doesn't work that way. It doesn't matter how much insurance you have, you cannot be admitted to a hospital without meeting specific admission criteria. This usually requires a life-threatening illness, where a medical intervention requires services available only at the hospital. Failing to meet these criteria, the only potential option is a short-term nursing home stay. However, nursing homes can come with some financial liability to the patient or their family.

The third squad is an 88-year-old white female who was brought in from home. She has increasing weakness, diarrhea, and abdominal distention. She looks like a beach ball that's about ready to explode. She has no bowel sounds, and she's not responding very well either. I order some lab, but a film will tell the story.

I see a 17-year-old white male with fever, cough, sore throat, congestion, body aches, and diarrhea. The parents didn't want to go out in the weather to see their doctor. They usually go to the Mecca (a nearby city). Doctors in this town are not good enough for them the rest of the time, but when it's more convenient to stay in town, they come to my ER. I do a strep and influenza screen that are both negative. He's got a virus. I give him some symptomatic medicines and send him on his way.

Our balloon patient has a sigmoid volvulus. This is a relatively common problem in the elderly. Their colon becomes floppy and redundant. The distal most part of the colon isn't very well tethered, and can twist onto itself, producing a bowel obstruction. This frequently requires that the bowel be resected. Regardless, it's a surgical problem, so after a phone call it's someone else's problem.

Our lady with the diarrhea we give some fluids. Her lab is fine. She just has a garden-variety stomach bug. It's likely to get better over the next couple of days. There is no real reason to admit the patient. I coordinate with the patient's doctor and we decide to try to get the patient in a nursing home for a while. This is going to involve some expense for the patient and her family. They just about go through the roof about this. In the end, they decide to take her back home rather than incur uncovered expenses.

With many of these folks I really wonder about the underlying motivation of the family. What I've frequently found is that grandma or grandpa often has "some resources," social security, a pension, etc, that the family have control of while the recipient is in the home. If they go to the nursing home, these funds usually wind up being used to pay for the nursing home care. It's definitely a case of secondary gain. Now if grandma winds up in the hospital, that's paid for by Medicare, and doesn't involve direct financial liability. So obviously, the family would always rather have their "loved one" admitted to the hospital.

12:00 PM

Boy, it's turning into a real social work day! Our fourth squad is a 95-year-old white male brought after having a "spell." Apparently, he was staring off into space, and didn't respond for a few minutes. He's a demented little old guy who's pleasantly confused, and has no real complaints. The possibility of stroke is brought up, and I wind up obligated to prove there isn't one. I do a routine stroke work-up, and it's pretty well normal. Then the real story comes out. It seems that this guy's caretakers went on vacation yesterday, and it's expected that with the reported symptoms, that he will be kept in the hospital till they get back. I think not! In the end, I send him back home, and make a lot of people upset. We are not a babysitting facility. At $1000-1500 per hospital-day, it would be cheaper to send this guy first class on a World vacation tour. Once again, if he's that much of a problem, they need to consider nursing home, and not the Emergency Department.

2:00 PM

Finally, some down time…

4:45 PM

Well, the offices are closing, so folks are starting to filter in.

First we have a 27-year-old white female, a patient of doctor NONE, with two weeks of cough and chest pain. Of course she's s smoker, 2 packs a day. That's a given. And it's an emergency today. She's got a bit of viral bronchitis, and it's treated symptomatically.

Second we have a 27-year-old white male with an alleged "migraine" headache. He's getting to be quite the frequent flyer. He's very whiney, and insists on a narcotic. Not! I give him the usual, and the nurses shuffle him out the door.

Third is a 15-year-old white male who split open his eyebrow in a basketball mishap. He tried to do something with a butterfly Band-Aid, but it's not working very well. I slap in a few stitches, and he's on his way.

6:00 PM

Fourth, we're back to our pediatric clientele. It's a 16-month-old white female with a fever for a day. No Tylenol, no Motrin, it's an emergency. Everything is normal. The kid has a little virus, and guess what? She needs some Tylenol or Motrin.

Fifth is a 40-year-old white male with a fever, cough, and headache for a day. Of course he's a two pack a day smoker since he was nine, and he wouldn't think of getting a flu shot. He's got influenza, and so I put him on Tambiflu (an influenza antiviral). None of these influenza antivirals are very effective, but folks want to walk out with the cure. So there you go. It might knock a day or so off his illness, and there's a pretty good chance he'll wind up with vomiting or diarrhea for his troubles (common side effects).

Sixth is an 84-year-old white male with intermittent abdominal pain for the last two weeks. It's apparently worse tonight. He's rolled up in a ball, and moaning. His exam is unremarkable except for some diffuse abdominal tenderness. I have the nurse start some intravenous fluids, give him a whiff of Demerol (a narcotic), and start our routine abdominal pain work-up. I do a knee-jerk cardiac evaluation, just because of his age. We'll see.

Meanwhile, I see our seventh patient of the evening. It's a 4-year-old white male who's had some intermittent abdominal cramping, and "red" stools. The mom is sure he's bleeding out into his bowels, but the picture just doesn't jive. Here he is, just smiling up at me, and happy as a clam. His exam is completely normal. His stool is reddish, but tests negative for blood. More commonly, this is due to these kids drinking red Cool-Aid, or something else with red dye in it. At the worst, this kid might have one of the gut bugs going around, but this can be treated supportively.

Our eighth patient turns into something of a surprise. This is a 37-year-old white female who had been in a fender bender a couple of weeks before, and has had a persistent headache. She had had a complete evaluation immediately after the accident, including a head scan. Everything was normal. She did have several minutes during the accident where she lost consciousness. This is likely a post concussion headache. I'm faced with my repeat visit rule, and that is to always look harder when someone comes back to an Emergency Room for a repeat visit. I have her zipped off to CT to rescan her head, and then I wait…

In the meantime, I see our ninth patient of the evening. It's a 31-year-old white male with fever, cough, and body aches for two days. He also is a smoker, about a pack a day. He's very dramatic, and acts like he's dying. His exam is normal, but he puts on a good act. I check him for influenza, but the test is negative. I finally hit on his agenda, and it's that he wants a work release. I really didn't need the entertainment! I give him what he wants and send him on his way.

Tenth is 4-year-old white female who ran into a wall and split her lip. It's really a pretty nasty split through the full thickness of the lip. This is a repair that I will not do, especially in a girl. It's of cosmetic importance, and thus the liability (and litigation) risk is huge. I call the local facial surgeon, and pass it off to him.

Double whammy! Our grandpa with the belly pain has very positive cardiac enzymes, and our car wreck victim has a fractured skull. So our belly guy's having a unusual presentation of a heart attack, and our headache lady could be having a bleed into her brain. Both require immediate attention.

Our 84-year-old has a pretty normal looking EKG, so it's probably not a real big heart attack. I start a range of cardiac protective medicines, and call his regular doctor to try and pass him off quickly so I can take care of my other potentially critical patient. I let him know that I have another patient with a potential brain bleed, and that I need to have him take over his patient right away. It just doesn't seem to register with this doctor. He goes on and on wanting the smallest minutia on his patient's case, and then wants to argue with me that the cardiac enzymes aren't high enough to be a heart attack. I just about loose my cool. There's no way that the patient's going home, so the doc just needs to come and take care of his patient. After moaning and complaining for perhaps 10 minutes, he finally gives the nurse admission orders, and we get the patient upstairs.

Well we don't have neurosurgical capabilities at our facility, so I start lining things up for my other patient. I call the on-call trauma center and chat with their neurosurgeon. He tells me that, given the location of the fracture, the lack of observed blood on the CT, and the elapsed time since the injury, it is unlikely that there is a significant bleed in progress. He's very pleasant, and volunteers to accept the patient in transfer to check her out and verify that nothing threatening is in progress. Done! She is out of here. Ten minutes later I get her on a squad, and on her way. Whew...

I see our 4-year-old with the lip laceration after the surgeon is finished with her. He did a very nice job, but it took him the better part of an hour. That is more time than I could ever spend on a lip repair. I would get so far behind...

Then we're back to the more mundane. I see a 15-year-old white male who twisted his ankle. It's just sprained, and he goes home in an air-splint.

I also see an 8-month-old hispanic boy who had vomited once this evening. He's smiling at me and seems most interested in playing with my stethoscope. Maybe he's got the gut bug, if anything at all, but all it needs is supportive treatment.

The rest of the evening is pretty boring. I get all my charts dictated. It's the end of the month, and I'm going on vacation for ten days. It's about time...Sunny Florida is calling my name.

And I am out of here...

12:00 AM

Epilogue

"Much more ado about nothing..."

And so ends another month in the ER...

It was a month in the winter and, as anticipated, it brought with it a little different patient mix, as well as a number of different patient issues than we get during the summer months. This is a good thing, or at least I like to think so. I imagine that another month of just the same old stuff would be pretty boring to readers out there.

I've tried to stay pretty much true to form with realism. As I've eluded previously, I loathe the drama and hype that medicine and emergency medicine is usually afforded in the popular media. I feel this does a disservice to all involved. The public gets a fantasy view of medicine that reinforces a range of stereotypes. The same is true of our young folks who are considering a career in medicine. It's all made so much more exciting and dramatic than it really is.

I must admit that both of my books paint a rather irreverent picture of medicine. But let's be honest a minute. Who provides health care services in this country? They're just regular people, with a broad cross-section of values and experiences. As such, this includes the altruistic, the greedy, and everything in between. There are good doctors and bad doctors, just as there are good patients and bad patients. They don't all go around with a sign on their foreheads to identify what camp they belong to.

As a user of medical services you really need to be an intelligent and appropriate user. As a provider, or potential provider, of medical services you really need to have a realistic understanding of what's involved.

I hope that those of you who have read this book have found it useful. From others in the emergency medicine field that I have talked with over the years, my experiences are really pretty typical hospital facilities across the country. Some are better, and some are worse.

Emergency medicine is a necessary evil. It can be exciting or unpleasant, but in the end, it's a job that someone has to do.

The Author

"Such a deal..." (an inside joke—Thanks Julie!)

Well I guess I should say something about myself, if only because it makes such an unusual story. I grew up mostly in small towns in the Pacific Northwest in the 60's and 70's. I was a nerdy kind of guy who spent a lot of time in the library. I graduated high school early, and went to a small private college in my home state. Shortly after my seventeenth birthday, I started out working on a multiple major in Chemistry, Physics, Biology, Mathematics, and Economics.

After pursuing my ambitious multiple major for a time, I became anxious to get out of school and into the "real world". I was closest to completing a pure physics degree, and began directing my energies towards that end. It had occurred to me that I didn't know what a person could do, job wise, with a degree in physics, so I went to the chair of the physics department and asked his advice. His response in a nutshell was, "Well (pause), you could go to graduate school..."

It was shortly after this that my growing disillusionment gelled and, in the manner of the young and stupid, I dropped out of school. Unfortunately when you're nineteen, it doesn't matter how bright you are, you were pretty well unemployable back in the mid-70's.

I decided to go into the military, and enlisted in the United States Air Force. What I discovered is that slave labor is not a lot of fun. I looked to see if there was any Air Force education programs that I could get involved with in order to get back on track with my future. I wanted to get out of the enlisted ranks, and given that I still had something over three years of obligation that I still owed, a commissioning program seemed my best bet. Unfortunately I was told I didn't qualify as my last semester of college was such a shambles that it just killed my GPA. This left me in something of a quandary as to what to do next.

One thing I found I was able to do in the military was take advanced placement tests (CLEP, DANTES, ACT, and the like). These were free of charge for an Airman on active duty, and so I took them all. Over a 6-8 month period I accrued something over 100 semester hours in college credit via examination. With this, in addition to the 110 semester hours I had from College, I felt that it should be enough to get some kind of degree. I contacted several colleges, including the one I had previously attended, to see what options I had available. I was told invariably that I had to complete the last 36 odd semester hours on-campus. "Really stupid", I thought. I knew there had to be a better way.

I combed the nation for a college that catered to non-traditional students and found two. Both acted as credit banks to put together college credit from other institutions. I applied to both simultaneously. The one that responded quickest required that I complete additional 12 semester hours of senior level coursework or above. The other took forever to reply.

I enrolled as an unclassified student in a graduate program in Health Sciences that was available on the Air Force base where I was stationed. I completed the required work in about 5 months. In the end, I graduated with a Bachelor of Science in General Studies, and applied to OTS (Officer Training School).

Simultaneously with my OTS application, I applied for training in the fields of Missile Maintenance or Space Systems. I had grown up during the space race, had dreamed of being an astronaut, and felt that this would be a path close to that aspiration. I was told that because I had had calculus in college that I was instead going to be a

Communications Electronics Officer. It seems they don't get many folks who've completed calculus.

I spent 4 months in Officer Training School and was commissioned a Second Lieutenant in the Air Force at the age of twenty-one. I then spent 8 months in Communications Electronics School, plus an additional 4 months in Communication Computer School.

Throughout my time in the military, I never really did anything that required calculus. This must have something to do with the classic oxymoron about military intelligence, but it's hard to say.

I spent a total of 7 years in the military playing computer geek, before leaving to seek my fortune at the age of twenty-seven. During that time, the Air Force spent a tremendous amount for me to attend a wide range of military and commercial schools. I have estimated that I spent 3-4 years of my military stint in one school or another.

Towards the end of my time in the military I became interested in construction, and founded a construction company. A partner and I built houses in our spare time for about three years. This was a poor time for the construction industry. We worked a lot, but didn't make much for our efforts. It was an interesting experience, but perhaps not the best use of my time.

After the military, I went to work as a computer consultant for a DOD contractor. I did this for about 5 years. This was my transition from military computer geek to corporate computer geek.

Way back in High School I had thought of going into Medicine. This thought had recurred during the time that I was taking the graduate courses in health sciences before my commissioning. I had talked about possibly going to Medical School all along the way, but hadn't taken any definitive steps.

At twenty-eight, I found myself single and unattached. I had spent the better part of ten years talking about how I wanted to go to Medical School, and I felt I needed to either get on with it or forget it.

I spent two years repeating the pre-medicine basics while getting my financial house in order. I applied to the local medical school, and surprisingly to me, I was accepted immediately.

I spent the next four years in medical school, and managed to graduate with distinction. I was actually interested in Pathology as a path to genetics research (This was something I developed an interest in along the way. I see it as the future of medicine, but that's another story entirely). Unfortunately, there was an untimely surplus of folks wanting to be Pathologists, and so I wound up in my first fallback position, internal medicine (adult medicine).

While I was in my residency I moonlighted in several Emergency Departments around the area, and found that I liked it better than internal medicine. (Actually it was a bit more than JUST moonlighting. I was working so many hours at so many Emergency Departments, that I was making more than most of the staff physicians in my internal medicine training program.) It is noteworthy that the vast majority of emergencies in an Emergency Department are adult medical emergencies, and so internal medicine was not such a bad match.

There were no emergency medicine residencies locally available, and so I arranged for additional training in pediatrics, obstetrics, and the like to round out my formal adult medicine training. I completed my (enhanced) internal medicine residency, and have worked exclusively in emergency medicine since. To date I've worked almost exactly five years in the field.

Since residency, I have spent a year and a half of my spare time building a house (a flashback to my construction days) for my family. I then spent another year and a half completing a MBA (This was motivated both by an interest in investing to obtain financial independence, as well as in anticipation of perhaps founding a biotechnology company down the road). Through this I've maintained an interest in genetics and gene therapy, and will start a formal Ph.D. program in molecular biology and molecular genetics in about a year from the date of this writing. I will likely leave clinical medicine at that time, hopefully in advance of that 7-year burnout period I mentioned earlier.

And now for a bit of update…As I write this, my original book in this series "Hot Summer Nights: A Month in the ER" has just been release online. I've also gotten my web site up and going: *www.dr-s-md.com*. It has an associated email facility: *mail@www.dr-s-md.com*. I'm on track with everything else. I'm tossing around whether to work on an online Masters Degree in Computer Science in what free time I have (ha ha, can you say obsessive-compulsive?). I'm thinking that all the rest of this is going to monopolize my time for a couple more months at least. I'm a go for a Ph.D. program in the summer, so I want to get all the big stuff behind me.

So where do these medical tidbits go from here? It just depends. If I get enough positive feedback from my readers, I will consider other reality-based medicine topics. So, I leave it in your capable hands.

It's been interesting…

Dr. S